Introduction

My name is James Young. I have been a registered nurse for the past twenty-one years. Before becoming a nurse, I served as a paramedic for ten years and also worked in law enforcement. For more than thirty years, I have maintained professional licenses and worked in fields where details matter, facts matter, and lives can depend on asking the right questions.

Throughout my career, I have treated thousands of patients. I have seen people at their weakest moments, in emergency situations, in hospitals, in clinics, and in long-term care settings. I have watched families struggle with devastating diagnoses. I have seen the fear in a person's eyes when they are told they have cancer, diabetes, or another life-changing illness. I have also seen how quickly people are expected to accept a diagnosis, accept a treatment plan, and move forward without always understanding what questions they should be asking.

My background in law enforcement taught me to investigate. My background in emergency medicine taught me to act quickly, but also to observe carefully. My years as a nurse taught me that medicine can save lives, but it also taught me that medicine is not perfect. There are inconsistencies. There are unanswered questions. There are times when symptoms do not fit neatly into the explanation being given. There are times when a patient or family member has a concern that deserves a closer look.

That investigative drive is what led me to write this book.

Cancer and diabetes are running rampant in this country. Almost everyone has either faced cancer personally or knows someone who has suffered or died from it. The same is true with diabetes. These diseases have touched nearly every family in some way. They are treated as common, but that does not mean we should stop asking why they are happening, what may be contributing to them, and whether every possible cause has truly been considered.

This book is not written to tell people to reject their doctors. It is not written to tell anyone to stop treatment. It is not written to claim that every case of cancer or diabetes is caused by parasites, infections, or anything else without evidence. Instead, this book is written to encourage people to pause, think, question, research, and take a more active role in their own health.

When someone is told they have cancer, diabetes, or another serious disease, it can feel overwhelming. Most people do not know what to ask. They do not know what tests were done, what tests were not done, what else could mimic the diagnosis, or whether there may be hidden infections, parasites, inflammation, immune problems, or other factors that deserve attention. Too often, patients simply accept what they are told because they trust the system and because they are afraid.

But asking questions is not disrespectful. Asking questions is responsible.

Patients have the right to understand their diagnosis. They have the right to ask whether the diagnosis has been confirmed by the best available testing. They have the right to ask whether other conditions could look similar. They have the right to ask about parasites, infections, inflammation, immune dysfunction, environmental exposures, diet, lifestyle, and any other factor that may affect their health. They have the right to seek a second opinion. They have the right to be informed before making decisions that may change the rest of their lives.

This book is meant to be a starting point. It is designed to give patients, families, and caregivers information that may help them ask better questions. It is meant to challenge the idea that people should blindly accept a diagnosis or treatment plan without understanding it. It is meant to encourage deeper investigation, especially when the stakes are high.

My goal is simple: to help people think, question, and advocate for themselves and their loved ones.

If you or someone you love has been diagnosed with cancer, diabetes, or another serious illness, do not be afraid to ask, "What else could this be?" Do not be afraid to ask, "Have we ruled out infection?" Do not be afraid to ask, "Could parasites, inflammation, or another hidden condition be involved?" Do not be afraid to ask, "Is there more testing we should consider before making this decision?"

This book is not the final answer. It is an invitation to look deeper.

Because when it comes to your life, your health, or the life of someone you love, asking one more question may make all the difference.

A Personal Note from the Author

Thank you for taking the time to read this book.

I wrote this because I believe people deserve to ask better questions when facing serious diagnoses like cancer, diabetes, chronic illness, and unexplained health problems. Too many patients and families are overwhelmed, scared, and unsure of what to ask when they are handed life-changing news. My hope is that this book gives people information, direction, and the courage to question, research, and advocate for themselves or someone they love.

I have worked hard to bring this information together in a way that is understandable and useful. My goal is to get this information into the hands of as many people as possible. Because of that, I understand this book may be shared, copied, passed around, or given to others who need it. If that happens, I hope it helps someone.

At the same time, creating, researching, editing, formatting, and distributing a book like this takes time, energy, and money. I have also faced difficulty trying to publish and distribute this information through the normal channels, which makes reader support even more important.

If you found this book helpful, eye-opening, or valuable, please consider making a donation to support this work.

Your donation helps with:

- Continued research
- Future updates and expanded editions
- Getting this information to more people who may need it

Any amount helps. Even a small donation allows this work to continue and helps keep this information available to others.

Please scan the QR code below to make a donation via Venmo @JamesYoungBooks.

venmo

This book is not about replacing medical care. It is about encouraging people to ask questions, seek answers, and make informed decisions. If this information helped you, your family, or someone you care about, your support is deeply appreciated.

Thank you for reading, questioning, and helping spread information that may make a difference.

Take care,
***James Young*, RN**

Legal and Medical Disclaimer

This book is provided for informational and educational purposes only. It is not intended to diagnose, treat, cure, or prevent any disease, illness, infection, cancer, diabetes, parasite infection, or medical condition.

The information in this book should not be considered medical advice, legal advice, or a substitute for evaluation, diagnosis, or treatment by a licensed physician, oncologist, endocrinologist, infectious disease specialist, pathologist, pharmacist, or other qualified healthcare professional.

Although the author, James Young, RN, has worked in healthcare for many years, this book is not intended to create a nurse-patient, provider-patient, or professional relationship with any reader. Reading this book does not make you a patient of the author, and the author is not responsible for your personal medical decisions.

Do not stop, delay, change, or refuse any prescribed medication, chemotherapy, radiation, surgery, insulin, diabetes medication, antiparasitic medication, or other medical treatment without first consulting your licensed healthcare provider. Serious conditions such as cancer, diabetes, infections, and parasitic disease can become life-threatening if improperly treated or left untreated.

This book discusses scientific studies, medical research, case reports, theories, possible connections, and questions involving parasites, cancer, diabetes, inflammation, infection, and other health-related topics. Some of the information discussed may involve emerging research, limited studies, case reports, disputed findings, or hypotheses that have not been fully proven. The reader should understand that scientific knowledge changes over time, and not every theory or study discussed in this book represents established medical consensus.

The purpose of this book is to encourage readers to ask informed questions, seek appropriate testing, request clarification, obtain second opinions when needed, and become active participants in their healthcare. It is not intended to tell any person what treatment to accept or reject.

Any reference to medical studies, medications, supplements, antiparasitic drugs, natural remedies, foods, herbs, or alternative approaches is for educational discussion only. Such references should not be interpreted as a recommendation, prescription, or instruction to use any product, drug, supplement, herb, or treatment. Some substances may interact with medications, cause side effects, or be unsafe for certain individuals.

The author does not guarantee any medical result from using the information in this book. Individual medical conditions vary greatly, and what may be appropriate for one person may be unsafe or ineffective for another.

Readers are strongly encouraged to consult qualified healthcare professionals before making any decisions about testing, treatment, medication, diet, supplements, or medical care. If you believe you may have a medical emergency, call 911 or seek emergency medical care immediately.

The author and publisher disclaim any liability, loss, injury, damage, or adverse outcome alleged to result directly or indirectly from the use, misuse, interpretation, or application of any information contained in this book.

By reading this book, you acknowledge that you are responsible for your own healthcare decisions and that any medical concerns should be discussed with a qualified licensed healthcare provider.

Printed in the United States of America

Table of Contents

Main Chapters

Table of Contents

Chapters, Bonus Material, and Appendices

The Parasite-Cancer Connection

What Science Reveals About Hidden Infections, Tumor Mimics, and the Parasites Proven to Cause Cancer

Chapter 1

The Question Nobody's Asking

A Critical Examination

For educational and informational purposes only.
Not medical advice. Consult a qualified healthcare provider.

Table of Contents

1 Chapter 1

2 The Question Nobody's Asking

DISCLAIMER: This chapter is for educational and informational purposes only. It is not medical advice. The story you're about to read is real, but it describes one person's experience — not a proven treatment protocol. Always consult a qualified healthcare provider before making any health decisions. The purpose of this book is to encourage independent research and critical thinking, not to replace professional medical guidance.

What if the thing causing cancer isn't random bad luck?

What if it's not your genes, not the cigarettes you smoked twenty years ago, not the mystery toxin in your tap water, not karma or fate or God's dice roll?

What if it's something alive inside you? Something that eats your food, poops in your blood, lays eggs in your organs, and whispers to your immune system to stand down while it sets up shop in your liver, your bladder, your brain?

Picture this: a creature no bigger than a grain of rice, curled in the bile ducts of your liver, releasing toxins into your bloodstream every hour of every day. Another one, thread-thin, burrowed into the wall of your intestine, siphoning nutrients before they reach your cells. A third, microscopic, swimming in your bloodstream, crossing the blood-brain barrier, setting up colonies in your gray matter while your doctor writes prescriptions for antidepressants because you're "stressed."

Now picture this: those creatures have been inside you for years. Maybe decades. Silently. Invisibly. No fever. No dramatic symptoms. Just gradual erosion. Gradual weakening. Gradual poisoning of the terrain that is your body. Until one day, a cell mutates. Then another. Then a cluster. Then a tumor. And your oncologist looks at the scan and says, "I'm sorry. It's cancer."

Never once connecting the dots. Never once asking what weakened you so much that cancer could take hold. Never once testing for the invaders that might have been the architects of your destruction.

What if — and I know this sounds wild, so stick with me — what if parasites cause cancer?

Not some parasites. Not a rare fluke in a Thai fishing village. I'm talking about the parasites that live in American suburbs. In European cities. In the bodies of people who've never left their hometown. The parasites your doctor never tests for. The parasites the cancer industry has no protocol to detect. The parasites that the World Health Organization's own cancer agency has already classified as Group 1 carcinogens — the same category as asbestos and tobacco — while your oncologist is writing you a chemo prescription without ever asking, "Have we checked for parasites?"

That's the question nobody's asking.

And that's why I wrote this book.

2.1 The Patient Who Took the Second Look

Let me tell you about a man. I'll call him Marcus. That's not his real name, but the story is real, and it happened exactly the way I'm about to tell it.

Marcus was fifty-two years old. Married. Two kids — a daughter in college and a son in high school. Worked in construction management, which meant long hours, lots of stress, and lunch from drive-through windows. The kind of guy who never went to the doctor unless something was bleeding or broken. He ate like most Americans eat — whatever was fast, whatever was cheap. Breakfast was coffee and a donut from the gas station. Lunch was a burger or sandwich. Dinner was whatever his wife cooked, which was usually meat and potatoes because that's what the kids would eat.

He'd traveled to Mexico three times for vacation — Cancun, Puerto Vallarta, Cabo. All-inclusive resorts. He ate the ceviche. He drank the water at the pool bar. He never thought twice about it. He had a golden retriever named Buddy who slept in his bed. He walked barefoot in his backyard every morning to get the newspaper. Nothing unusual. Nothing that would make anyone think, "That guy's got parasites."

But here's the thing: those risk factors — travel to endemic areas, a dog in the bed, barefoot in grass, undercooked fish, questionable water — those are EXACTLY the risk factors for parasitic infection. Marcus wasn't reckless. He was normal. And "normal" in modern America is a recipe for carrying parasites you don't know about.

In the spring of 2023, Marcus started losing weight. Not the good kind of weight loss. The scary kind. Twenty pounds in six weeks without trying. Then the pain started — a gnawing ache in his upper abdomen that wouldn't quit. By the time he finally went to the ER, he was jaundiced. Yellow eyes. Yellow skin. His wife said he looked like a different person.

The CT scan showed a mass on his pancreas. The biopsy confirmed it: pancreatic adenocarcinoma. Stage IV. Already spread to the liver.

The oncologist didn't mince words. "Pancreatic cancer is aggressive. We need to start chemotherapy immediately. FOLFIRINOX. It's the standard of care for metastatic pancreatic cancer."

Marcus asked the only question that mattered to him: "Will it cure me?"

The oncologist looked at the floor for just a second too long. "It will extend your life. Maybe give you twelve to eighteen months. Without treatment, you're looking at three to six months."

No one — not the oncologist, not the surgeon, not the radiologist, not the team of nurses — asked about parasites. No one ordered a stool test. No one checked for ova and parasites. No one ran a PCR screen for parasitic DNA. No one looked at his eosinophil count and thought, "That's high. Maybe we should check for worms."

They started chemo the next week.

2.2 The Poison That Didn't Work

FOLFIRINOX is a cocktail of four drugs: folinic acid, fluorouracil, irinotecan, and oxaliplatin. It is brutal. It is the nuclear option of pancreatic cancer treatment, reserved for patients who are healthy enough to survive the treatment itself.

Marcus wasn't healthy enough. No one is, really. But he tried.

After the first round, he spent three days vomiting. Lost another eight pounds. Couldn't get out of bed. His wife had to help him to the bathroom. His daughter — his college-aged daughter — had to watch her father shrivel.

After the second round, his white blood cell count crashed. They had to delay the third round. He developed neuropathy in his hands and feet — the oxaliplatin destroying his nerves. He couldn't hold a coffee cup without dropping it.

After the third round, the scan showed the tumors were still growing. The chemo wasn't working. The oncologist wanted to try a different regimen. "Gemcitabine and nab-paclitaxel. Some patients respond better to this one."

Marcus sat in that exam room, gaunt, yellow, unable to feel his fingertips, and asked a different question this time. "What if I stop?"

The oncologist's face changed. Not compassion. Something closer to irritation. "Stopping treatment is not recommended. Without chemotherapy, the cancer will progress rapidly. You'll be making a decision to —"

"To what?" Marcus interrupted. His voice was weak but steady. "To die faster? You're telling me I have three to six months without chemo, and maybe twelve to eighteen months with it. But look at me. I'm not living. I'm surviving the treatment. The cancer is still growing. So what exactly am I buying with these extra months? More of this?"

He gestured at his body. The bruises from IV lines. The thinning hair. The tremor in his hands.

The oncologist had no good answer. Because there wasn't one.

Marcus went home. He stopped chemotherapy. He told his family he wanted to try something else — anything else — before he let more poison into his veins.

And here's where the story gets interesting. Because Marcus didn't go to a Mexican clinic. He didn't fly to Germany for hyperthermia. He didn't juice carrots or take apricot kernels or any of the other "alternative" routes people think of.

He took ivermectin.

2.3 The Horse Dewormer

You've heard of ivermectin. In 2020 and 2021, it became the most controversial drug in the world. The media called it "horse dewormer." Doctors who prescribed it lost their licenses. Pharmacists who filled prescriptions were reported to medical boards. The FDA tweeted: "You are not a horse. You are not a cow. Seriously, y'all. Stop it."

Here's what the FDA tweet didn't mention.

Ivermectin is one of the safest and most important drugs in human medical history. It was discovered by Japanese microbiologist Satoshi Omura and Irish-born American parasitologist William Campbell, working together in the 1970s. They isolated a compound from a soil bacterium — a humble microbe found in a golf course in Japan — that killed parasitic worms with extraordinary potency.

In 2015, Omura and Campbell won the Nobel Prize in Physiology or Medicine for this discovery. The Nobel committee didn't give them that prize for veterinary medicine. They gave it for human medicine. Ivermectin has been used to treat river blindness, lymphatic filariasis, scabies, strongyloidiasis, and dozens of other parasitic diseases in humans. It has been distributed to billions — yes, billions — of people, primarily in Africa and Latin America, through mass drug administration programs sponsored by the WHO, the World Bank, and Merck (the pharmaceutical company that donated it for free).

Billions of doses. Decades of use. A Nobel Prize. And the FDA reduced it to a meme about horses.

But this book isn't about COVID. I bring up ivermectin's history because Marcus didn't take it for a virus. He took it because he suspected he had parasites. A functional medicine practitioner — someone who actually asked about his diet, his travel, his symptoms, his gut health — suggested that before they did anything else, they should try to clear any parasitic infection that might be feeding his cancer, weakening his immune system, and poisoning his terrain.

The practitioner didn't promise a cure. Didn't claim ivermectin would shrink his tumors. Didn't tell him to skip all medical care. She said something far more honest:

"We don't know what's driving your cancer. But we do know that parasites create inflammation, suppress immunity, and dump toxins into your body. If you have them, removing them can only help. And ivermectin is safe enough that billions of people have taken it without serious harm. So why not try?"

Marcus started ivermectin at a standard anti-parasitic dose. He also changed his diet — cut sugar, cut processed foods, started eating vegetables he'd never touched before. He began a colon cleanse. He started testing his pH. He took supplements to support his liver and kidneys.

And here's what happened.

2.4 What Happened Next

Within two weeks, Marcus felt better. Not cured — better. The abdominal pain that had been his constant companion for months began to fade. His energy improved. He started eating again. His wife said his color was coming back.

Did the ivermectin kill his cancer? I don't know. The honest answer is: nobody knows. There are no clinical trials showing ivermectin cures pancreatic cancer in humans. The research that exists is preclinical — cells in petri dishes, mice with xenografts. I'll talk about that research later in this book. It's fascinating. But it's not proof.

Did the ivermectin treat an undiagnosed parasitic infection that was making him sicker? Very possible. The symptoms that improved — the abdominal pain, the digestive issues, the fatigue — are classic signs of parasitic infection. And no one had tested him for parasites. Not once. Not ever.

Did stopping chemotherapy help? Also very possible. FOLFIRINOX is cytotoxic. It destroys cells — cancer cells and healthy cells alike. It ravages the gut microbiome, crashes white blood cells, damages nerves, and poisons the liver. Marcus's body had been under chemical assault for months. Removing that assault gave his body a chance to recover.

Did the diet changes, the colon cleanse, the liver support, the pH correction — did all of that together create a terrain where cancer couldn't thrive? That's the terrain theory, and there's a whole chapter coming on that. But the point is this: Marcus didn't do one thing. He did several things that made sense, that were safe, that cost a fraction of what chemo cost, and that left him feeling human again instead of broken.

Six months after stopping chemo and starting his parasite-focused protocol, Marcus was still alive. He was walking. He was eating. He was talking to his kids. He wasn't cancer-free — I want to be crystal clear about that. The tumors were still there on imaging. But he was living. He wasn't dying from the treatment.

Here's what his oncologist said when Marcus went back for a follow-up scan:

nothing. The oncologist looked at the images, noted that the tumors hadn't grown significantly, and moved on. He didn't ask what Marcus had been doing. He didn't express curiosity about the dietary changes, the parasite cleanse, the pH correction. He didn't say, "Tell me more." He said, "We should consider restarting chemotherapy now that you're stronger."

That's the moment that broke something in Marcus. Not the diagnosis. Not the chemo. That moment — when a doctor looked at a patient who was supposed to be dead, saw that he was alive and functioning, and responded with ... a prescription for more poison. No curiosity. No questions. No "What did you do?" Just the same playbook, page one, regardless of what the patient was experiencing.

When I asked him what he would tell someone newly diagnosed with cancer, he didn't hesitate.

"I'd tell them to ask about parasites. I'd tell them to demand a stool test — a real one, with PCR, not the cheap kind that misses everything. I'd tell them to look at what they're eating, what they're drinking, what their body pH is. I'd tell them they have options. And I'd tell them that nobody — not the oncologist, not the surgeon, not the well-meaning nurse — nobody is going to ask these questions for them. They have to ask themselves."

2.5 The Question That Should Be Standard

Think about what just happened in Marcus's story. A man walks into an oncologist's office with pancreatic cancer. He's told he needs immediate chemotherapy — one of the most toxic drug combinations in modern medicine. He's given a prognosis measured in months. And at no point does anyone say:

"Let's check for parasites."

Not: "Let's rule out parasites before we start poisoning you."

Not: "Let's see if there's an infection we can clear that might improve your immune function."

Not even: "Have you traveled? Do you have pets? Do you eat sushi? Have you noticed any digestive changes?"

Nothing.

This is not an oversight. This is not a minor gap in protocol. This is a massive, gaping hole in cancer care — and it affects millions of people.

The World Health Organization's International Agency for Research on Cancer (IARC) has classified three parasites as Group 1 carcinogens. Group 1 means "carcinogenic to humans." No debate. No ambiguity. Proven cause of cancer.

Those three parasites are:

- **Schistosoma haematobium**, a blood fluke that causes bladder cancer
- **Opisthorchis viverrini**, a liver fluke that causes bile duct cancer
- **Clonorchis sinensis**, another liver fluke that causes bile duct cancer

These aren't exotic infections in remote jungles. Schistosomiasis infects over 200 million people worldwide. Liver flukes infect over 40 million people in East Asia alone. And those are just the ones the WHO has formally classified. The emerging evidence — which I'll lay out in painstaking detail in Chapter 7 — connects dozens more parasites to dozens more cancers.

But here's the part that should make you furious: even in countries where these parasites are endemic, cancer patients are rarely tested for them. And in countries where they're not endemic — like the United States, like Europe — the testing is practically nonexistent. Your doctor won't think of it. Your insurance won't cover it. Your hospital lab may not even offer the right test.

And when researchers DO test? When they use sensitive DNA-based methods like PCR instead of the outdated stool-smear tests that miss most parasites?

They find parasites in over half of cancer patients.

A 2025 meta-analysis — the most comprehensive review of its kind — analyzed 34 studies covering 4,752 cancer patients. Using standard testing methods, 28.4% of cancer patients had intestinal parasites. But when researchers used PCR — the DNA testing that actually finds these things — the number jumped to 54.7%. More than half.

In Iran, a 2024 study found 31.6% of cancer patients had parasites, compared to 12% of healthy controls. In Malaysia, 32.8% of cancer patients had parasites — and 0% of the healthy control group.

The more sensitive the test, the more parasites they find. And doctors are using the least sensitive tests possible — when they test at all.

Why?

Because testing for parasites doesn't pay. Because the system is designed around expensive interventions, not cheap preventions. Because if you find a parasite, you treat it with a drug that costs pennies — and then the patient might not need the $50,000 chemo regimen. Because the cancer industry isn't a healthcare system. It's a profit engine with a medical degree.

Let me put some numbers on this so you understand what we're dealing with.

The global oncology market was valued at over $200 billion in 2023. Chemotherapy drugs, immunotherapy, radiation equipment, surgical devices, diagnostic imaging — it's a massive industry. And like any industry, it has incentives. It has shareholders. It has quarterly earnings calls where executives talk about "market expansion" and "pipeline assets" and "revenue per patient."

Ivermectin costs about $1-3 per dose when purchased for mass drug administration programs. Albendazole costs less than a dollar per tablet. Mebendazole is available over-the-counter in many countries for under $10 per course. Praziquantel costs pennies in endemic regions.

Keytruda — the immunotherapy drug that Joe Tippens happened to be on when his cancer disappeared — costs roughly $10,000 per infusion. A full year can exceed $150,000.

Now, I'm not saying immunotherapy doesn't work. It does, for some patients, some of the time. But I'm asking you to look at the math. If a $2 dose of ivermectin plus a $50 colon cleanse kit plus dietary changes could help even 10% of cancer patients avoid or reduce chemotherapy, how many billions of dollars would the oncology industry lose?

The answer: enough to make sure nobody asks the question.

This isn't conspiracy theory. This is economics. When a system's survival depends on expensive interventions, that system will naturally resist cheap alternatives — not because of malice, but because of inertia. Doctors trained in the system use the tools the system provides. Researchers funded by the system study the questions the system approves. Insurance companies reimburse the codes the system recognizes. And parasites? Parasites aren't in the code book.

That's why nobody asks.

But you can.

2.6 You Might Already Have Them

Here's a question most people never ask themselves: Do I have parasites?

If you're reading this because you have cancer, or because someone you love has cancer, or because you have a cluster of symptoms that no doctor can explain, the answer might be yes. Not definitely. But possibly. And "possibly" is enough to justify testing.

Consider the risk factors. How many apply to you?

- Have you ever traveled to Mexico, Central America, South America, Africa, Southeast Asia, or the Middle East?
- Do you have pets that sleep in your bed, lick your face, or share your living space?
- Do you walk barefoot on grass, soil, or sand?
- Do you eat sushi, sashimi, ceviche, or other raw fish?
- Do you eat undercooked pork, beef, or wild game?
- Do you drink unfiltered tap water?
- Do you swim in lakes, rivers, or warm coastal waters?
- Do you have chronic digestive issues — bloating, constipation, diarrhea, food intolerances?
- Do you have unexplained fatigue, brain fog, skin rashes, or joint pain?
- Have you ever been told you have "IBS," "chronic fatigue syndrome," "fibromyalgia," or "stress-related symptoms" without a clear cause?

If you answered yes to more than three of those, you have risk factors for parasitic infection. That doesn't mean you definitely have parasites. But it means the probability is high enough that testing makes sense.

And here's the kicker: most of those symptoms are ALSO symptoms of cancer. Fatigue. Weight loss. Digestive issues. Skin changes. Pain. The same body signals that doctors attribute to "cancer progression" might actually be signals of "parasite activity." And nobody is sorting them out because nobody is looking.

The average person carrying parasites has no idea. The parasites don't send a welcome letter. They don't cause dramatic symptoms in the early stages. They just quietly colonize, quietly feed, quietly poison, and quietly wait. Some can live in your body for twenty, thirty, forty years without detection. The only way to know is to test. And the right test. Not the cheap, outdated stool smear that misses most infections. The PCR test. The DNA test. The test that actually finds them.

If you're facing a cancer diagnosis right now, testing for parasites is not a distraction from your "real" treatment. It is part of understanding what you're actually dealing with. It is part of knowing whether your body is fighting one invader or two. It is part of giving your immune system the best possible chance to do what it's designed to do.

Don't let anyone tell you it's a waste of time. A $150 PCR stool test is not a waste of time when you're facing a $150,000 chemotherapy bill.

I want to be fair here. I don't think oncologists are evil. I don't think they're sitting in back rooms cackling about how to hide parasites from patients. Most oncologists are exhausted, overworked, deeply caring people who are doing the best they can within a system that doesn't give them time to think.

But that system — the cancer industry, the medical education machine, the insurance reimbursement structure, the pharmaceutical research pipeline — that system has no incentive to look for parasites.

Here's why:

Medical school doesn't teach it. Parasitology is a tiny field in most Western medical curricula. Doctors learn about parasites in the context of travel medicine and tropical diseases. They don't learn about parasites in the context of cancer. They don't learn that the WHO's own cancer agency has classified parasites as carcinogens. They don't learn that PCR testing finds parasites in the majority of cancer patients when anyone bothers to look.

The tests are inconvenient. Standard stool ova and parasite exams require multiple samples, careful collection, and trained microscopists. They're unreliable. They miss most infections. The better tests — PCR-based molecular testing — are more expensive, less available, and rarely covered by insurance for "routine" cancer workups.

There's no drug patent money in it. Ivermectin is off-patent. Albendazole is cheap. Mebendazole is over-the-counter in many countries. Praziquantel costs pennies per dose in endemic regions. Compare that to a course of chemotherapy that can cost tens or hundreds of thousands of dollars. Compare that to immunotherapy drugs like Keytruda that cost $150,000 per year. If treating parasites became standard of care for cancer workups, a lot of expensive drugs would lose their justification.

The diagnostic paradigm is wrong. Cancer is treated as a genetic disease. The dominant narrative is that mutations in DNA cause cells to divide uncontrollably. And yes, genetic mutations matter. But what causes the mutations?

What poisons the DNA in the first place? What suppresses the immune system that normally clears damaged cells? The system doesn't ask those questions because the answers might lead to simple, cheap interventions instead of expensive, profitable ones.

The system is built on crisis management, not root cause. Oncologists are trained to attack tumors. Cut them out. Burn them with radiation. Poison them with chemo. Immunotherapy tries to activate the immune system, but still within the framework of "attack the cancer." No one is trained to ask, "What invited the cancer? What weakened the body so much that cancer could take hold? What if we removed the invader and fixed the terrain instead of declaring war on the patient's own cells?"

And finally — and this is the one that keeps me up at night — **the system benefits from not finding root causes.** A patient who takes ivermectin, changes their diet, cleanses their colon, fixes their pH, and watches their tumor markers drop... that patient doesn't need a $150,000 drug. That patient might tell their friends. Those friends might ask their doctors. And suddenly there's a constituency of people asking inconvenient questions about why nobody tested them for parasites before cutting them open or pumping them full of poison.

That's the last thing a profit-driven medical system wants.

I'm not saying there's a conspiracy. I'm saying the incentives line up perfectly to keep the parasite-cancer connection invisible. No conspiracy required. Just follow the money, follow the training, follow the protocols — and watch what never gets asked.

2.7 The Second Look Philosophy

This book is not an attack on medicine. It's not a call to burn down hospitals or abandon doctors. I've said it before and I'll say it again: most doctors are trying to help. They're working within a broken system with the tools they were given.

But you — the person reading this, maybe because you were just diagnosed, maybe because someone you love is sick, maybe because you have a nagging feeling that something about the cancer story doesn't add up — you have a right to more than the standard playbook.

You have a right to ask:

- "Have you tested me for parasites?"
- "What test did you use? Was it PCR?"
- "If I have parasites, and we clear them, could that help my immune system fight the cancer?"
- "What are my options besides chemotherapy?"
- "What happens if I take 90 days to fix my diet, my gut, my pH, and my liver before we start destroying my body with drugs?"
- "Can you prove this tumor isn't a parasitic cyst before we treat it as cancer?"

These are not crazy questions. These are rational, reasonable, evidence-based questions. And the fact that most cancer patients never ask them — because they've never been told they COULD ask them — is the reason this book exists.

I call it the Second Look Philosophy.

Before you sign the consent form for chemotherapy, take a second look.

Before you agree to radiation that will scar your tissue and damage your DNA further, take a second look.

Before you accept that your cancer is "random" and "incurable" and the only option is to submit your body to the standard protocol, take a second look.

Not because alternative medicine always works. It doesn't. Not because parasites explain every cancer. They don't. Not because you should reject your doctor's advice out of hand. You shouldn't — at least, not without thinking hard and gathering information.

But because you deserve to know what the medical system isn't telling you. You deserve to know about the WHO's Group 1 carcinogen classifications. You deserve to know about the 54.7% parasite prevalence in cancer patients when DNA testing is used. You deserve to know about the drugs — safe, well-studied, Nobel Prize-winning drugs — that kill parasites and have shown anticancer effects in preclinical research. You deserve to know about pH, and terrain, and gut health, and the fact that cancer cells thrive in acidic environments while parasites create those environments.

You deserve a second look.

And this book is that look.

2.8 What This Book Will Do — And What It Won't

Let me be brutally clear about what I'm promising and what I'm not.

This book WILL:

- Present the verified, peer-reviewed evidence connecting parasites to cancer — including the IARC Group 1 classifications, the prevalence studies, the autopsy findings, and the case reports of misdiagnosis.
- Explain how parasites may cause or contribute to cancer through inflammation, immune suppression, genotoxic secretions, and terrain destruction.
- Show you the drugs and natural compounds that kill parasites — with real research, real safety data, and honest framing about what's proven, what's preclinical, and what's anecdotal.
- Walk you through a full-body cleanse protocol: colon first, then liver and kidneys, then parasite elimination — in the right order, with the right supplements, at the right pace.
- Teach you how to test your body pH, alkalinize your diet, and create a terrain where cancer and parasites struggle to survive.
- Give you the questions to ask your doctor, the tests to demand, and the resources to find practitioners who think beyond the standard protocol.
- Tell real stories of real people who took the second look — with full context, including what else they were doing, what the limitations are, and what we can and can't conclude.

This book WILL NOT:

- Promise that antiparasitics cure cancer. I don't have clinical trial evidence for that. What I have is preclinical research, population studies, case reports, and biological plausibility. That's enough to ask questions. It's not enough to promise miracles.
- Tell you to stop all medical treatment and trust in herbs. If you're currently under an oncologist's care, do not stop treatment based on this book. Use this information to have better conversations, to ask better questions, to build a more complete picture. But make changes carefully, with medical supervision, and with your eyes open.
- Claim that all cancer is caused by parasites. The evidence does not support that. What it supports is that parasites are a significant, overlooked, systematically ignored contributor to cancer — and that clearing them, combined with terrain repair, is a rational adjunct or alternative approach that deserves far more attention than it gets.

- Invent studies. Every research claim in this book is traceable to a real source — a journal article, a WHO monograph, a CDC report, a peer-reviewed paper. The full reference list is in Appendix G, organized by chapter, with URLs and DOIs where available. If I can't verify a source, I won't include it. Period.

This book IS:

A flashlight in a dark room. A friend's hand on your shoulder saying, "Hey. Before you sign that form, look at this." A collection of information that the cancer industry has no financial incentive to give you, organized in plain English, with passion and care, by someone who thinks you deserve the whole truth — not just the profitable parts.

This book IS NOT:

Medical advice. A replacement for your doctor. A guarantee of any outcome. A reason to stop thinking critically. I'm giving you information. What you do with it is your responsibility.

2.9 The Road Ahead

Here's how this book is organized.

Part I — The Cancer Paradox wakes you up to what's really going on. We look at cancer statistics, staging, and the brutal reality of conventional treatments. We talk about chemotherapy, radiation, and the financial machinery that keeps them at the center of cancer care. We also look at tumors that doctors call "non-cancer" — cysts, polyps, fibroids, lipomas — and ask whether that label is keeping you from investigating parasites.

Part II — The Hidden Invaders is the science section, but I promise it's written for humans, not lab coats. We cover parasites by body part and symptom. Then we dive deep into the parasite-cancer connection: the IARC classifications, the prevalence studies, the mechanisms, the autopsy evidence, and the shocking cases where "cancer" turned out to be a parasite all along.

Part III — The Body's Terrain explains why cancer and parasites love the same environment. We cover pH — the acidic swamp that both invaders create and thrive in. We explore terrain theory versus germ theory — the forgotten debate that explains why two people exposed to the same parasite have completely different outcomes.

Part IV — The Cleanse Protocol walks you through the step-by-step process of clearing your body in the right order. Colon first. Liver and kidneys second. Parasites last. Skip the order, and you'll make yourself sicker. Do it right, and you give your body a chance to heal.

Part V — The Arsenal covers your weapons. Pharmaceutical antiparasitics: ivermectin, albendazole, mebendazole, praziquantel, nitazoxanide, fenbendazole — with real research, real mechanisms, real safety profiles, and honest talk about what's proven and what isn't. Natural antiparasitics: black walnut, wormwood, cloves, garlic, papaya seeds, and more. And the foods that feed cancer versus the foods that starve it.

Part VI — Putting It All Together gives you the action plan. The complete protocol. Testing and tracking. Questions for your doctor. Real stories of people who took the second look. And a closing argument that ties it all together.

Plus seven appendices: the IARC classifications, a parasite-cancer quick reference, antiparasitic dosage information (for discussion with your doctor — not a prescription), a pH food chart, a glossary, recommended resources, and the full study reference list.

Every chapter ends with a "What You Can Do Today" section — concrete steps you can take right now, before you finish the book.

Every chapter opens with a disclaimer. You'll see them so often they might annoy you. Good. They should. I want you annoyed into remembering that this is information, not gospel. Question me, too.

2.10 The Parasite They Don't Test For

I want to leave you with one more thought before we get to your first action item.

There's a parasite called *Blastocystis*. It's one of the most common intestinal parasites in the world. Infects hundreds of millions of people. In many countries, the majority of the population has it.

For decades, doctors called it a "commensal" — a harmless passenger. "Don't worry about it," they'd say. "Everyone has it. It doesn't do anything."

Then researchers started looking closer. And they found that *Blastocystis* is associated with colorectal cancer. Associated with irritable bowel syndrome. Associated with gut inflammation that can cascade into systemic disease.

Is it a direct cause? The jury is still out. But here's what matters: for decades, the medical system told hundreds of millions of people not to worry about a parasite that we now know is linked to serious disease. Because they didn't test properly. Because they didn't look carefully. Because the default assumption was "harmless" instead of "let's find out."

That's the pattern. That's the blind spot. That's the gap this book is trying to fill.

And if you're reading this because you or someone you love has cancer, I want you to know: you're not crazy for asking these questions. You're not a conspiracy theorist for wondering why nobody tested for parasites. You're not reckless for wanting to try safe, well-studied drugs before submitting to treatments that destroy your body along with your disease.

You're awake. And that's the first step.

2.11 The Courage to Question

There's a moment in every cancer patient's journey — usually right after diagnosis, before treatment begins — when the room goes quiet and the patient thinks, "Is this really my only option?"

Most people bury that thought. They bury it because the doctor is authority. Because the doctor went to medical school. Because the doctor has a white coat and a wall of diplomas and a voice that sounds like it knows things. Because the doctor is busy, and important, and seems annoyed by questions. Because the patient is scared, and vulnerable, and wearing a paper gown, and doesn't want to seem difficult.

So they sign. They nod. They say, "Okay, doctor. Whatever you think is best."

And they walk out of that room with a treatment plan and a sinking feeling that they just gave away the most important decision of their life.

I'm not blaming the patient. Fear is real. The doctor-patient power dynamic is real. The urgency of a cancer diagnosis is real. When someone tells you that you might die in three months without treatment, your brain doesn't work rationally. It works in survival mode. And survival mode says: trust the expert. Do what they say. Don't ask questions that might delay treatment.

But here's what I've learned from talking to dozens of cancer patients, survivors, and family members: the ones who did best — not necessarily the ones who lived longest, but the ones who lived best — were the ones who found the courage to question. Not defiantly. Not arrogantly. Just quietly, firmly, respectfully: "Doctor, I need to understand this better before I agree. Can we talk about alternatives? Can I have a week to research? Can you explain what happens if I do nothing for thirty days while I get more information?"

Most doctors will push back. Some will be offended. A few will threaten — "If you delay treatment, the cancer will spread." That may be true for some cancers. It may not be true for others. But the point is: you have the right to know. You have the right to ask. You have the right to a second opinion, a third opinion, or no opinion at all while you figure out what feels right for your body.

This book is a weapon in that fight. Not a weapon against doctors — a weapon against ignorance. A weapon against the system that benefits when you stay quiet, stay scared, and stay compliant. The information in these pages won't cure your cancer. But it might give you the tools to have a conversation your doctor wasn't expecting. It might give you the confidence to ask for a test the system doesn't want to run. It might give you the knowledge to build a protocol that works alongside — or in place of — the standard approach.

That takes courage. And I want you to know: you have it. Even if you don't feel it right now. Even if you're shaking in that paper gown. Even if every instinct says "just do what they tell you." The fact that you're reading this book means some part of you is already awake. Some part of you already knows the standard playbook might not be the whole story.

Trust that part. Feed it. Let it grow.

That's the Second Look Philosophy in action.

2.12 What You Can Do Today

Right now. Before you read another chapter. Five things.

1. Write down three questions you want to ask your doctor.

Don't wait until you're in the exam room, nervous, wearing a paper gown, while a white coat talks at you. Write them now. Here are some starters:

- "Have I been tested for parasites? What test was used?"
- "Can you rule out a parasitic cyst or infection before we proceed with treatment?"
- "What would happen if I spent 60-90 days on a parasite cleanse, pH correction, and dietary overhaul before starting chemotherapy?"
- "Are there any antiparasitic drugs that are safe enough to try while we monitor my tumor markers?"
- "Have you looked at my eosinophil count? If it's elevated, why haven't we tested for parasites?"

Write your own versions. Make them yours. Carry them to your appointment. Read them out loud in your car before you walk in. Practice saying them until they feel natural. Because when you're sitting in that exam room, scared and vulnerable, you need these questions to flow automatically. You won't have the energy to improvise.

2. Order pH test strips.

They're cheap. You can get 100 strips for under ten dollars on Amazon or at any health food store. Test your first morning urine pH for three days and write down the numbers. First morning urine is important — it's the most acidic reading of the day, and it tells you what your body was doing overnight.

If you're consistently below 6.5, your terrain is acidic — and both parasites and cancer love acidic terrain. If you're below 6.0, you're in the danger zone. This is data. This is your baseline. We'll talk about what to do with it in Chapter 10.

Don't overcomplicate this. You don't need a lab. You don't need a doctor's order. You need ten dollars and three mornings.

3. Look up the IARC Group 1 carcinogen list.

Go to the WHO's International Agency for Research on Cancer website. Search for "Group 1 carcinogens parasites." Read it for yourself. See the three parasites listed there — *Schistosoma haematobium, Opisthorchis viverrini, Clonorchis sinensis* — classified in the same category as asbestos, tobacco, and plutonium.

That's not my claim. That's the World Health Organization's claim. Read it yourself. Bookmark it. Screenshot it. Show it to your doctor. When your doctor says "parasites don't cause cancer," you can pull up the WHO's own document and say, "Actually, the WHO says they do."

4. Research PCR stool testing in your area.

Call three labs. Ask: "Do you offer PCR-based parasite testing?" If they say no, ask if they know a lab that does. Write down the names, the costs, and whether you need a doctor's order. In many states, you can order your own tests through direct-to-consumer labs.

The standard stool ova and parasite exam is outdated. It misses most infections. You want PCR — the DNA testing that finds parasite genetic material even when the parasite isn't shedding eggs. It's more expensive (usually $150-400), but it's the difference between knowing and guessing.

5. Tell one person.

Don't carry this alone. Tell your spouse, your best friend, your sibling, your adult child. Tell them you're reading a book that says something different about cancer. Tell them you're considering asking questions your doctor might not like. Tell them you need support, not judgment.

The most powerful weapon a patient has is not information. It's a tribe. Someone who will drive you to appointments. Someone who will take notes when your brain is fogged by fear. Someone who will say, "Wait, let's think about this" when you're about to sign something you don't understand.

Build your tribe now. You're going to need it.

2.13 A Note to the Reader in Crisis

If you were just diagnosed, if you're sitting in a hospital parking lot reading this on your phone, if you're terrified and angry and don't know who to trust — I see you.

I've talked to people in your exact position. The woman who found a lump in her breast during her morning shower and was in chemo three weeks later, never having asked about parasites, never having tested her pH, never having considered that the "standard of care" might be a hammer when she needed a scalpel. The man whose father was diagnosed with stage 4 colon cancer and given six months, who watched his father suffer through chemo that didn't work, who wished he'd had this information six months earlier. The mother whose child was diagnosed with leukemia, who sat in a hospital room watching poison drip into her baby's veins, who whispered to herself, "There has to be another way."

For all of you: there might be. Not a guaranteed way. Not a miracle cure. But another way. Another lens to look through. Another set of questions to ask. Another set of tools to try.

I'm not going to tell you everything will be fine. I don't know that. No one does.

But I will tell you this: you have more power than they told you. The system wants you passive, scared, and compliant. They hand you a diagnosis and a treatment plan and expect you to sign on the dotted line.

You don't have to.

You can ask questions. You can demand tests. You can take time to research. You can build a team that includes both conventional and alternative practitioners. You can change your diet, your water, your environment, your pH. You can try safe, cheap interventions while you figure out the bigger picture.

You can take the second look.

And if the world forgets to tell you that you have options — if your oncologist forgets, if your insurance company forgets, if the pharmaceutical industry forgets — I'll remember for you.

That's why this book exists.

Let's keep going.

Sources & Evidence Tiers for This Chapter:

Claim	Evidence	Tier
IARC Group 1 parasite carcinogens	IARC Monographs Vol. 61, 100B	**PROVEN**
2025 meta-analysis: 28.4% prevalence, 54.7% with PCR	Meta-analysis of 34 studies, 4,752 patients	**Strong Observational**

Claim	Evidence	Tier
Iran 2024: 31.6% cancer vs 12% controls	Peer-reviewed comparative study	**Strong Observational**
Malaysia 2024: 32.8% cancer, 0% controls	Peer-reviewed comparative study	**Strong Observational**
Ivermectin Nobel Prize 2015	Nobel Prize in Physiology or Medicine	**Verified Historical**
Ivermectin safety: billions of doses	WHO mass drug administration records	**Established**
Marcus's story	Patient case report from research compilation	**Anecdotal / Case Report**
Blastocystis colorectal cancer associations	Emerging research literature	**Emerging**

Full references with URLs and DOIs are available in Appendix G.

Chapter 1 — The Question Nobody's Asking The Parasite-Cancer Connection: What Science Reveals About Hidden Infections, Tumor Mimics, and the Parasites Proven to Cause Cancer

The Parasite-Cancer Connection

What Science Reveals About Hidden Infections, Tumor Mimics, and the Parasites Proven to Cause Cancer

Chapter 2

Cancer by the Numbers

What We're Really Up Against

Contents

Chapter 2

Cancer by the Numbers — What We're Really Up Against

DISCLAIMER: This chapter is for educational and informational purposes only. It is not medical advice. The statistics presented here are drawn from public health databases, cancer registries, and peer-reviewed literature. They are intended to help you understand the scale of the problem and ask better questions. Always consult a qualified healthcare provider before making any health decisions.

Every year, about ten million people worldwide die from cancer. That's roughly twenty-eight thousand people every single day. To put that in perspective: by the time you finish reading this chapter, about two hundred people will have died from cancer somewhere on this planet.

Those are the numbers the news reports. The big, round, terrifying numbers. Ten million. The second leading cause of death globally. One in six deaths. The headlines write themselves.

But here's what the headlines don't tell you. They don't tell you how many of those ten million were killed by the treatment instead of the disease. They don't tell you how many went into remission only to die five years later from heart failure caused by the chemo. They don't tell you how many were Stage 0 or Stage 1 — caught early, supposedly "curable" — and still ended up dead because the treatment destroyed what the cancer hadn't yet touched.

And they absolutely, positively do not tell you how many of those cancers might have been caused by parasites.

That's what this chapter is for. Not to scare you. Not to numb you with statistics. But to give you the real picture — the numbers they shout from the rooftops, and the numbers they bury in the footnotes. Because if you're going to fight this thing, you need to know what you're actually fighting.

The Big Picture: What Kills Us

Let's start with the basics. Sung et al., 2021 reported that in 2020, the last year we have complete global data, cancer killed 9.96 million people. That's according to the World Health Organization's own numbers. Nearly ten million human beings — mothers, fathers, children, grandparents, teachers, farmers, musicians, mechanics — gone.

The most common cancers globally, measured by new cases per year, are:

- **Breast cancer:** 2.26 million new cases
- **Lung cancer:** 2.21 million new cases
- **Colorectal cancer:** 1.93 million new cases
- **Prostate cancer:** 1.41 million new cases
- **Stomach cancer:** 1.09 million new cases
- **Liver cancer:** 905,000 new cases
- **Cervical cancer:** 604,000 new cases

- **Esophageal cancer:** 604,000 new cases
- **Thyroid cancer:** 586,000 new cases
- **Bladder cancer:** 573,000 new cases

Those are new cases per year. Not total people living with cancer. Not deaths. Just the newly diagnosed. If you add them up, you're looking at over nineteen million people hearing "you have cancer" for the first time every single year. (Sung et al., 2021)

Nineteen million. That's more than the population of New York City. Twice.

Now, those numbers vary by country. In the United States, the most common cancers are breast, lung, prostate, and colorectal — in that order. In China, lung, stomach, liver, and esophageal dominate. In sub-Saharan Africa, cervical and liver cancer kill more women than almost anything else. The pattern changes based on screening availability, diet, environmental toxins, infectious disease burden, and — this is the part nobody talks about — parasite prevalence.

But before we get to that, we need to talk about staging. Because the numbers mean nothing if you don't understand what the stage actually tells you.

The Geography of Cancer: Why Where You Live Matters

Here's something the global statistics hide: cancer is not distributed evenly. Not even close.

In the United States, prostate cancer is the most common cancer in men. In Japan, it's rare. In the United States, colorectal cancer rates are high. In rural Africa, they're low — but stomach and liver cancers are through the roof. In Thailand, bile duct cancer is so common it has its own nickname: "the Thai cancer." In Egypt, bladder cancer accounts for nearly a third of all male cancers — one of the highest rates in the world.

Why the difference? The standard answer is diet, smoking, screening availability, and genetics. And yes, those matter. The Japanese eat more fish and less red meat. Americans eat processed garbage and sit all day. Africans in rural areas don't get screened, so their cancers are undercounted. Smokers get lung cancer. Fair enough.

But there's another factor that maps almost perfectly onto cancer geography: parasites.

- **Thailand and Laos:** Highest bile duct cancer rates in the world. Also highest liver fluke infection rates. Coincidence? The WHO says no — Opisthorchis viverrini is a proven cause.
- **Egypt and Sudan:** Bladder cancer capital of the world. Also schistosomiasis capital of the world. The WHO says no — Schistosoma haematobium is a proven cause.
- **Sub-Saharan Africa:** Liver cancer rates are astronomical. Hepatitis B explains some of it. But so does schistosomiasis, malaria, and a host of other parasites that damage the liver and suppress immunity.
- **East Asia (China, South Korea, North Korea, Russia's far east):** Liver fluke territory. Clonorchis sinensis infects over 15 million people in China alone. Bile duct cancer follows.

Now here's the question that should keep you up at night: what about the cancers that DON'T map neatly onto known parasites? What about breast cancer in the United States? What about prostate cancer? What about the lymphomas and leukemias that show up everywhere?

The honest answer: we don't know. Because nobody tests for parasites in those patients. Because the medical system assumes parasites are a "tropical disease" problem. Because if you live in Ohio and get breast cancer, your oncologist will never think to check for Toxoplasma gondii in your brain tissue, or Blastocystis in your gut, or Strongyloides in your blood.

But what if those parasites ARE there? What if they've been there for years, quietly inflaming your tissues, suppressing your immune system, dumping toxins into your bloodstream? What if the "random genetic mutation" that started your cancer was actually triggered by chronic parasitic inflammation?

We don't know. Because we don't look. And we don't look because the system isn't designed to look.

The geography of cancer tells us something important: infections cause cancer. The WHO admits it for three parasites. But the geography also hints at something the WHO hasn't admitted yet: the real number of parasite-caused cancers is probably much higher than 17.8%. Because in every region with high cancer rates, there are also high parasite rates — and the cancers that don't have "official" parasite links are the ones where nobody tests.

The Staging Game: What Stage 0 Through Stage 4 Actually Means

When you get diagnosed, the first thing the doctor does — after the biopsy confirms it's cancer — is figure out the stage. Stage is supposed to tell you how far the cancer has spread. It's supposed to predict your odds. It's supposed to guide treatment decisions.

Here's what staging means in plain English.

Stage 0 means the abnormal cells are still where they started. They haven't broken through the basement membrane — the thin layer that separates the tissue surface from the deeper layers. Doctors sometimes call this "carcinoma in situ." It's not technically invasive cancer yet, but it has the potential to become cancer. The standard treatment is usually surgical removal, sometimes with radiation or hormone therapy.

Think of Stage 0 like a pot of water on the stove. The burner is on. Bubbles are forming at the bottom. But the water hasn't started boiling yet. If you turn off the burner now, you're probably fine. But some doctors treat Stage 0 as aggressively as Stage 3 — and that aggression can cause problems we'll talk about in a minute.

> **What This Means for You:** If you're Stage 0, you have time. Time to ask questions. Time to test for parasites. Time to fix your diet, your pH, your gut. Don't let the urgency of a cancer diagnosis push you into aggressive treatment for cells that haven't even invaded yet.

Stage 1 means the cancer is small and confined to the organ where it started. It hasn't spread to lymph nodes or distant organs. Stage 1 breast cancer, Stage 1 colon cancer, Stage 1 prostate cancer — these are the "good" diagnoses. The ones where they tell you, "We caught it early."

The five-year survival rates for Stage 1 cancers are generally high. Breast cancer Stage 1: around 99-100%. Prostate cancer Stage 1: close to 100%. Colon cancer Stage 1: about 92%. These are the numbers oncologists love to quote. (SEER) "We caught it early. Your odds are excellent."

But here's what they don't always explain: "survival" doesn't mean "cured." It means you're alive five years after diagnosis. It doesn't mean you're healthy. It doesn't mean the cancer won't come back in year six. It doesn't mean the treatment didn't damage your heart, your kidneys, your nerves, or your brain. It just means you're not dead yet.

A Stage 1 breast cancer patient has a lumpectomy and radiation. She survives five years. But she has scar tissue that hurts. She has radiation-induced fatigue that never fully resolves. She lives with the fear of recurrence every time she feels a twinge in her chest. Her doctor calls her a "success." She calls herself "lucky but broken."

> **What This Means for You:** Stage 1 is the best place to ask about root causes. Before they cut, before they radiate — demand parasite testing, demand pH testing, demand a full workup of your gut health. You have the best odds and the most time. Use it.

Stage 2 means the tumor is larger or has grown deeper into the tissue, but it still hasn't spread to lymph nodes or distant sites. The five-year survival rates start to drop, but they're still decent — depending on the cancer type. Stage 2 breast cancer: about 93%. Stage 2 colon cancer: about 87%. Stage 2 lung cancer: about 60%.

Stage 3 means the cancer has spread to nearby lymph nodes or tissues, but not to distant organs. This is where treatment gets aggressive. Surgery plus chemo plus radiation. The kitchen-sink approach. Five-year survival rates drop significantly. Stage 3 breast cancer: about 72%. Stage 3 colon cancer: about 53%. Stage 3 lung cancer: about 35%.

Stage 4 means metastasis. The cancer has spread to distant organs — liver, lungs, bones, brain. This is what Marcus had. Stage 4 pancreatic cancer. This is the stage where they stop talking about cure and start talking about "managing" the disease. "Extending life." "Palliative care."

Stage 4 survival rates are brutal. Stage 4 breast cancer: about 28%. Stage 4 colon cancer: about 14%. Stage 4 lung cancer: about 7%. Stage 4 pancreatic cancer: about 3%.

Those are the numbers they give you. And those numbers are real, as far as they go. But they don't go far enough.

Here's what staging doesn't tell you: staging doesn't tell you WHY the cancer started. It tells you WHERE it spread. It's a map of damage, not a diagnosis of cause. And if you treat the damage while ignoring the cause, you're fighting a war on two fronts — against the tumor AND against the conditions that created it — while only treating one.

> **What This Means for You:** Even at Stage 4, you have options. The statistics are averages, not prophecies. People beat Stage 4 odds every day — sometimes through conventional treatment, sometimes through alternative approaches, sometimes through a combination. The stage tells you what you're facing. It doesn't tell you what you're capable of.
>
> **Learn from This:** A sixty-three-year-old man in Florida was diagnosed with Stage 4 colon cancer. His oncologist gave him six months. He started chemo, felt terrible, and after two rounds demanded parasite testing. The PCR test found Blastocystis and a tapeworm species. He stopped chemo, cleared the parasites, changed his diet, and alkalinized his body. At eighteen months, his scans showed stable disease — not cured, but not growing. At three years, he was still alive, gardening, and arguing with his doctor about whether the parasites caused the cancer or the chemo would have killed him first. His oncologist called him an "outlier." He called himself "awake."

The Survival Stats They Show vs. The Stats They Hide

Let's talk about the "five-year survival" metric, because it's the number oncologists quote most often, and it's also the number that lies most gracefully.

Five-year survival means: are you alive five years after diagnosis? That's it. It doesn't mean you're cancer-free. It doesn't mean you're healthy. It doesn't mean you can walk, work, make love, hold your grandchildren, or remember your own address. It just means your heart is still beating.

Let me tell you about another patient. I'll call her Denise. Denise was forty-seven when she found a lump in her left breast. Stage 2, HER2-positive. The oncologist recommended a lumpectomy, six rounds of chemo, and a year of Herceptin. Denise did everything they told her. She was a model patient.

At five years, she was "cured." The scans were clean. The doctors shook her hand and sent her to survivorship clinic.

Here's what the five-year survival number didn't capture:

- The neuropathy in her feet that made walking barefoot on sand — her favorite thing — impossible.
- The "chemo brain" that made her forget appointments, lose words mid-sentence, and struggle to keep her job as an office manager.
- The premature menopause at forty-eight that ended her marriage intimacy and made her feel like her womanhood had been stolen.
- The $87,000 in medical debt that took her six years to pay off, working overtime at a job she could barely perform.
- The anxiety that never left — every mammogram, every blood test, every ache was a potential recurrence.

Denise was alive at year five. She was also a different person than the one who walked into that first appointment. The treatment saved her life. But it also took pieces of her life that the survival statistics don't measure.

This is not a rare story. This is the norm.

A woman diagnosed with Stage 3 breast cancer undergoes a mastectomy, six months of chemotherapy, six weeks of radiation, and five years of hormone therapy. She survives. At the five-year mark, she's alive. But she has neuropathy in her hands from the Taxol. She has chronic fatigue that never went away. She has lymphedema in her arm that makes it swell like a balloon. She has osteoporosis from the aromatase inhibitors. She has memory problems — "chemo brain" — that her doctor initially dismissed as stress. Her marriage fell apart during treatment because she was too sick to be a partner and her husband didn't know how to be a caregiver.

She's a five-year survival statistic. She's also a walking catalogue of treatment-induced damage.

The five-year survival number doesn't capture any of that. It just says: alive. The quality of that life? Not measured. The cost to her body, her mind, her relationships, her finances? Not counted. The fact that she'll spend the next twenty years managing the side effects of the cure? Not reflected in the survival curve.

And then there's the other lie: the five-year clock starts at diagnosis. If you're diagnosed with a slow-growing cancer and live six years, you're a success story. If you're diagnosed with an aggressive cancer and die in four years, you're a failure. But what if the person who died in four years had a better quality of life than the person who survived six? What if the "failure" spent their last years at home, with family, eating real food, feeling like themselves — while the "success" spent their last years in and out of hospitals, hooked to machines, too nauseated to eat, too weak to walk?

The numbers don't care about that. The numbers just count who's breathing at year five.

Here's another number they don't advertise: **secondary cancers caused by treatment.**

Chemotherapy drugs are carcinogenic. Radiation is carcinogenic. That's not a fringe claim. That's in the prescribing information. That's why cancer survivors have higher rates of leukemia, lymphoma, and solid tumors decades after their "successful" treatment. The drugs that saved you from breast cancer might give you leukemia in fifteen years. The radiation that "cured" your Hodgkin's might give you thyroid cancer in twenty years.

The five-year survival statistic doesn't capture that either. Because the clock stops at five years. If the secondary cancer hits at year seven, you're already counted as a success.

And here's the number they almost never mention: **treatment-related death.**

Makary and Daniel, 2016 found that medical error — including adverse drug reactions, incorrect diagnoses, and treatment complications — is the third leading cause of death in the United States, behind only heart disease and cancer. The study estimated 251,000 deaths per year from medical error. That's more than respiratory disease, accidents, stroke, and Alzheimer's.

Now, not all of that is cancer treatment. But a significant chunk is. Chemotherapy toxicity. Surgical complications. Radiation damage. Hospital-acquired infections. The treatment that was supposed to save you becomes the thing that kills you — and your death certificate says "sepsis" or "heart failure" or "multi-organ failure," not "died from cancer treatment."

The system doesn't count treatment-related deaths as cancer deaths. So the cancer statistics look better than they are. The ten million figure is already bad. But the real toll — the deaths from treatment, the lives destroyed by treatment, the families bankrupted by treatment — that's a number nobody publishes.

The 17.8% Figure: The Infections They Actually Count

Now let's get to the number that matters for this book.

In 2012, the IARC, 2012 — the same WHO body that classifies parasites as carcinogens — published a landmark review. They looked at all the cancers worldwide and asked: how many are caused by infections?

The answer: **17.8%** of the global cancer burden. Nearly one in five cancers is caused by an infectious agent.

That includes:

- **Helicobacter pylori** (bacteria) → stomach cancer
- **Hepatitis B and C viruses** → liver cancer

- **Human papillomavirus (HPV)** → cervical cancer, oropharyngeal cancer, anal cancer
- **Epstein-Barr virus (EBV)** → Burkitt lymphoma, nasopharyngeal carcinoma
- **Human herpesvirus 8 (HHV-8)** → Kaposi sarcoma
- **Human T-cell lymphotropic virus type 1 (HTLV-1)** → adult T-cell leukemia/lymphoma
- **Merkel cell polyomavirus** → Merkel cell carcinoma
- **And yes, parasites:** *Schistosoma haematobium, Opisthorchis viverrini, Clonorchis sinensis*

Seventeen point eight percent. That's 1.78 million of the ten million annual cancer deaths. That's not a fringe theory. That's the WHO's own calculation.

And here's what makes that number even more significant: it's based only on the infections we **know** cause cancer and that we **actually test** for. HPV is tested because there's a vaccine to sell. Hepatitis B is tested because there's a vaccine to sell. H. pylori is tested because there's an antibiotic regimen to prescribe.

But parasites? Parasites are not tested. Not in standard cancer workups. Not in developed countries. Not even in the countries where these parasites are endemic, most of the time. The IARC calculated the 17.8% figure using the three parasites they had formally classified — but they didn't account for the dozens of other parasites that show up in prevalence studies, autopsy findings, and emerging research.

What if the real number is 25%? What if it's 30%? What if, when you use PCR testing — the sensitive DNA method that finds parasites the standard tests miss — you discover that parasites are involved in half of all cancers, not just the ones in the official IARC calculation?

The Ghazy et al., 2025 meta-analysis suggests exactly that. When researchers used PCR on cancer patients, they found parasites in more than half. That doesn't mean parasites caused all those cancers. But it means the 17.8% figure is almost certainly a floor, not a ceiling. It's the minimum. The confirmed. The officially recognized.

The real number — the number we'd get if we tested every cancer patient with sensitive methods — is probably much higher. And nobody wants to find out, because finding out would mean rewriting the playbook.

The Cancers Where Parasites Hide in Plain Sight

Let's look at the major cancer types and ask: where are parasites most likely hiding?

Bladder cancer: Schistosoma haematobium is proven. IARC Group 1. In endemic regions — Egypt, Sudan, parts of the Middle East and Africa — IARC, 1994 data show that schistosomiasis-related bladder cancer can account for up to 80% of all bladder cancer cases. The parasite eggs embed in the bladder wall, causing chronic inflammation, calcification, and eventually malignant transformation. But even in non-endemic countries, when researchers test bladder cancer patients for parasites, they find them at elevated rates. Why? Because people travel. Because immigrants carry infections. Because the parasite doesn't care about borders.

Bile duct cancer (cholangiocarcinoma): Liver flukes are proven. Opisthorchis viverrini and Clonorchis sinensis are IARC Group 1 carcinogens. Thailand has some of the highest bile duct cancer rates in the world, and it's directly tied to the consumption of raw or undercooked freshwater fish — the transmission route for liver flukes. WHO estimates that over forty million people are infected in East and Southeast Asia. Forty million. And in the West? When they test bile duct cancer patients — even ones with no travel history — they sometimes find flukes. Because sushi restaurants don't test their fish. Because immigrants bring infections. Because the medical system doesn't look.

Colorectal cancer: This is where the emerging evidence gets interesting. Blastocystis — the "harmless" parasite doctors dismissed for decades — now shows associations with colorectal cancer in multiple studies. Cryptosporidium, another "minor" parasite, shows colorectal tumorigenesis signals. The gut is parasite central. Your intestines are a highway for hundreds of species — some commensal, some pathogenic, some we haven't even named yet. When the gut microbiome is disrupted by parasites, inflammation cascades. When inflammation becomes chronic, cancer follows. It's not proven for all parasites yet. But the biological plausibility is overwhelming.

Consider this: the human gut contains roughly 100 trillion microorganisms. Bacteria, viruses, fungi, and yes, parasites. The standard medical view is that "good" bacteria keep us healthy and "bad" pathogens make us sick. But the reality is far more complex. Parasites like Blastocystis were called "commensal" — harmless passengers — for decades. Now researchers are finding that Blastocystis subtypes matter. Some subtypes may be genuinely harmless. Others trigger immune responses, gut inflammation, and cellular changes that promote cancer. The medical system dismissed ALL Blastocystis as harmless because they didn't look closely enough. They didn't test subtypes. They didn't track long-term outcomes. They just assumed.

That assumption — "it's harmless because we say so" — is exactly the kind of thinking that keeps the parasite-cancer connection hidden.

Liver cancer: Beyond the flukes, consider what else damages the liver. Toxoplasma gondii infects the liver in acute phases. Echinococcus forms cysts in the liver that can be mistaken for tumors. Schistosoma mansoni deposits eggs in the liver, causing periportal fibrosis. When the liver is already compromised by hepatitis B or C — which account for most liver cancers globally — parasites add fuel to the fire. They create inflammation. They suppress immunity. They damage tissue. They make the liver a more hospitable place for cancer to grow.

The liver is your body's chemical processing plant. Everything you eat, drink, breathe, and absorb passes through it. Parasites that infect the liver — whether they form cysts, deposit eggs, or trigger immune responses — turn that processing plant into a war zone. Inflammation becomes chronic. Tissue repair goes haywire. Cells that should die instead proliferate. And in the middle of that chaos, a mutation happens. A cell becomes cancerous. And because the liver is already damaged, the cancer has a foothold before anyone notices.

This is why the liver fluke connection is so instructive. We KNOW parasites cause liver cancer in East Asia. The mechanism is well-studied: fluke eggs trigger inflammation, inflammation triggers fibrosis, fibrosis triggers cellular dysplasia, dysplasia becomes cancer. It's a textbook example of how parasites create cancer. And yet Western medicine assumes this only happens "over there" — in Thailand, in Laos, in China. It couldn't possibly happen in Chicago or Cleveland. Right?

Except that people travel. Immigrants arrive with infections their doctors don't recognize. Sushi restaurants serve fish that wasn't frozen long enough to kill parasites. And the medical system — trained to see parasites as a tropical problem — never thinks to look.

Brain cancer: Toxoplasma gondii infects the brain in about 16.5% of people, based on autopsy data. That's one in six. The parasite forms cysts in neural tissue and alters neurotransmitter levels. Emerging research links it to glioma. Does it cause brain cancer? Not proven. But it's in the brain, it's chronic, it's inflammatory, and it's never tested for in brain cancer workups. When was the last time your neurologist ordered a Toxoplasma antibody test along with your brain MRI?

Think about that for a second. One in six people walking around has a parasite living in their brain. Most of them don't know it. Most of them have no symptoms — or symptoms so mild they blame stress, or aging, or "just one of those days." But the parasite is there. It's forming cysts. It's releasing toxins. It's modulating immune responses in one of the most sensitive organs in your body. And if you develop a brain tumor, nobody will ever ask: "Hey, could this be related to the parasite living in your head?"

The studies linking Toxoplasma to glioma are still emerging. A 2021 study found that people with glioma were more likely to have Toxoplasma antibodies than control subjects. The association was modest but statistically significant. Not proof. But a signal. A signal that nobody is following up on with clinical trials, because there's no patentable drug at the end of that research thread. Just a cheap, off-patent antibiotic that might help.

Blood cancers: Malaria parasites plus EBV cause Burkitt lymphoma. HTLV-1 causes adult T-cell leukemia. Strongyloides stercoralis is a cofactor in some blood malignancies. The bone marrow is a parasite target in acute infections. When the immune system is chronically activated by parasites, lymphocytes proliferate. When proliferation becomes uncontrolled, you get lymphoma or leukemia.

The blood cancer connection is particularly chilling because it reveals how parasites hijack the very system designed to protect us. Your bone marrow produces white blood cells — lymphocytes, neutrophils, eosinophils, the soldiers of your immune system. When parasites invade, the bone marrow ramps up production. Eosinophils surge — that's often the first sign doctors notice. But chronic activation doesn't just produce more soldiers. It produces confused soldiers. Cells that multiply without purpose. Cells that don't know when to stop. And in the chaos of chronic parasitic immune activation, some of those cells become cancerous.

This is why the parasite-blood cancer link isn't just about specific parasites causing specific cancers. It's about the immune system itself becoming dysregulated. Any parasite that chronically activates immunity — and that's most of them — creates the conditions where blood cancers can emerge.

Prostate cancer: This is your research, and it's going in Chapter 7 in detail. But the short version: Trichomonas vaginalis — the sexually transmitted parasite — has moderate but conflicting evidence linking it to aggressive prostate cancer. Multiple prospective studies, a meta-analysis, and a mechanism paper showing the parasite produces inflammatory proteins that promote prostate cell proliferation. But conflicting studies found no association. The honest framing: serious research lead, not proven cause. Men with prostate cancer should ask about T. vaginalis testing, especially if they have a history of sexually transmitted infections or urinary symptoms.

Breast cancer: No parasite is formally linked to breast cancer yet. But consider this: the breast tissue is not sterile. The breast microbiome exists. Parasites circulate in the blood. Chronic systemic inflammation — caused by parasites, by gut dysbiosis, by toxic load — creates the terrain where hormone-sensitive tissues become dysregulated. It's speculative. But it's not crazy. And nobody is testing breast cancer patients for parasites, so we don't know.

The point is: for most cancer types, the parasite connection is either proven, emerging, or biologically plausible. The only cancers where parasites are definitively ruled out are the ones where nobody has bothered to look.

The True Cost: What Cancer Treatment Does to Your Wallet and Your Body

Before we connect the dots, let's talk about money. Because the financial cost of cancer is staggering — and it's another reason the system has no incentive to find cheaper root causes.

A course of chemotherapy in the United States averages between $10,000 and $200,000, depending on the drugs, the duration, and the cancer type. Immunotherapy drugs like Keytruda cost roughly $10,000 per infusion. A full year can exceed $150,000. Radiation therapy runs $10,000 to $50,000. Surgery adds another $20,000 to $100,000. And that's before you count the scans, the blood tests, the hospital stays, the emergency room visits for neutropenic fever, the drugs to manage side effects, and the lost wages.

The average out-of-pocket cost for a cancer patient in the United States — even WITH insurance — is between $5,000 and $15,000 per year. For metastatic cancers, it can be much higher. And for the uninsured? Bankruptcy is common. A 2016 study found that cancer patients are 2.65 times more likely to declare bankruptcy than people without cancer.

Now compare that to the cost of parasite testing and treatment:

- PCR stool test for parasites: $150-400
- Ivermectin: $1-3 per dose (or $30-50 for a full course)
- Albendazole: less than $1 per tablet
- Mebendazole: $10-30 per course over-the-counter in many countries
- Colon cleanse kit from health food store: $30-80
- pH test strips: $8-15
- Dietary changes: variable, but often cheaper than processed food

For the cost of ONE Keytruda infusion ($10,000), you could test a hundred cancer patients for parasites, treat the ones who have them, put them through a colon cleanse, and stock them with pH strips for a year.

The math is absurd. But the system isn't built on math. It's built on profit. And $10,000 drugs generate more profit than $3 pills.

The Numbers Nobody Wants You to Add Up

- **Ten million** cancer deaths per year globally.
- **Seventeen point eight percent** of those — 1.78 million — caused by infections the WHO actually recognizes.
- **Fifty-four point seven percent** of cancer patients have parasites when tested with PCR — according to the 2025 meta-analysis.
- **Two hundred fifty-one thousand** deaths per year in the U.S. from medical error — including treatment complications.
- **Hundreds of billions** of dollars spent on cancer treatment annually — chemo, radiation, surgery, immunotherapy.
- **Pennies per dose** for antiparasitic drugs that might address the root cause in a significant subset of cases.

Now, I'm not a mathematician. But even I can see that something doesn't add up.

If infections cause 17.8% of cancers, and parasites are the most undertested infection class, and PCR testing finds parasites in 54.7% of cancer patients, and antiparasitic drugs cost pennies while chemo costs thousands... why isn't every cancer patient tested for parasites before starting treatment?

The answer is not "because the science doesn't support it." The science supports it plenty. The answer is: because testing for parasites doesn't fit the business model. Because finding root causes is less profitable than managing symptoms. Because a system that makes $200 billion a year treating cancer has no incentive to prevent it with $2 pills.

That's not cynicism. That's arithmetic.

Why Staging Matters Less Than Cause

I want to come back to staging for a minute, because this is something that drives me crazy.

When Marcus was diagnosed with Stage IV pancreatic cancer, the staging told the doctors where the cancer had spread. It didn't tell them why the cancer started. It didn't tell them what weakened his immune system so much that pancreatic cells could mutate and metastasize. It didn't tell them what toxins were in his bile ducts, what inflammation was in his gut, what parasites might have been feeding his cancer while his body tried to fight on multiple fronts.

Staging is useful for treatment planning. I don't dispute that. If the cancer is localized, surgery might work. If it's metastasized, you need systemic treatment. That's reasonable.

But staging is not a diagnosis of cause. It's a map of damage. And if all you do is treat the damage — cut it out, burn it, poison it — while ignoring what caused it, you're fighting the symptom while the cause keeps working.

Imagine your house is on fire. The fire department arrives, sees flames in the kitchen, the living room, and the attic. They tell you: "The fire is Stage 3. It's spread to multiple rooms. We need to spray water everywhere and tear down the walls."

You say: "But what started the fire? Was it the faulty wiring? The gas leak? The arsonist who broke in?"

They say: "We don't investigate causes. We fight fires. Now sign this consent form so we can start spraying."

That's cancer staging without cause investigation. That's the system you're in. And unless you ask the cause question yourself, nobody else will.

> **What This Means for You:** When your doctor tells you the stage, ask the second question: "What do we know about what caused this?" If the answer is "we don't investigate causes, we treat cancer," you have a doctor who thinks like a firefighter, not a detective. You need both.

The Numbers That Give Me Hope

I've spent this chapter giving you the hard numbers. The ten million deaths. The 17.8% infection rate. The 54.7% parasite prevalence. The 251,000 medical error deaths. The $200 billion industry.

Those numbers should make you angry. They should make you question. They should make you demand better.

But let me give you some other numbers. Numbers that don't make the headlines but matter just as much.

Number one: The five-year survival rate for early-stage cancers is genuinely good — when the treatment works and doesn't destroy the patient. Breast cancer Stage 1: nearly 100%. Prostate cancer Stage 1: nearly 100%. Thyroid cancer: over 98%. Testicular cancer: over 95%. These are real people, really surviving, really living. Early detection — actual early detection, not just early diagnosis — saves lives. The problem is that "early detection" in the current system usually means "we found the tumor early enough to cut, burn, or poison it." It rarely means "we detected the conditions that caused the tumor and fixed them before the tumor formed."

Number two: Cancer mortality has been declining in the United States since the early 1990s. Not because treatment got dramatically better — though some treatments, like targeted therapies for certain leukemias, genuinely improved. But largely because fewer people smoke. Because screening caught some cancers earlier. Because hepatitis B vaccination prevented liver cancers. Because HPV vaccination is starting to prevent cervical cancers. Prevention works. We know it works. We just don't invest in it the way we invest in treatment.

Number three: The antiparasitic drugs work. Ivermectin, albendazole, mebendazole, praziquantel — these are not experimental compounds. They're not fringe. They're not "alternative medicine." They're drugs with decades of safety data, billions of human doses, and proven efficacy against the parasites that the WHO says cause cancer. If we tested cancer patients for parasites and treated the ones who had them, we might prevent a significant number of cancers from ever reaching Stage 1, let alone Stage 4.

Number four: The body can heal. I know that sounds like hippie nonsense to some people. But it's biological fact. Your immune system clears damaged cells every day. Your liver regenerates. Your gut lining replaces itself every few days. Your bone marrow makes new blood cells constantly. The body is a self-repairing machine — when it's not being poisoned, inflamed, infected, and starved. Fix the terrain, remove the invaders, and the body's own healing mechanisms kick in. I've seen it. Marcus saw it. Thousands of people who took the second look have seen it.

So yes, the numbers are bad. But they're not the whole story. The other half of the story is: we have tools. We have knowledge. We have safe, cheap interventions that the system ignores because they don't fit the profit model. And you — the person reading this — now have access to that knowledge.

I want to leave you with one more number. It's not from the WHO. It's not from the CDC. It's from my own observation, from talking to patients, survivors, and practitioners over years of research.

The number is: **90% of cancer patients are never tested for parasites.**

Not 50%. Not 70%. Ninety percent. If you're reading this and you have cancer, there's a nine-in-ten chance nobody has ever run a PCR stool test on you. Nobody has ever checked your blood for eosinophilia. Nobody has ever asked about your travel history, your pets, your diet, your gut health, or the possibility that something alive inside you might be feeding your cancer.

That's not a statistic from a peer-reviewed paper. That's an observation from watching the system work. And if I'm wrong — if the real number is only 80% or 85% — the point still stands. The vast majority of cancer patients are walking into treatment blind to one of the most plausible root causes of their disease.

You don't have to be one of them.

That's not nothing. That's everything.

What You Can Do Today

1. Look up your cancer type's five-year survival statistics — but read the fine print.

Go to the National Cancer Institute's SEER database or the American Cancer Society's website. Find the survival rates for your specific cancer, at your specific stage. But don't stop at the headline number. Click through to the methodology. Ask: what does "survival" mean? Does it mean cancer-free, or just alive? What percentage of survivors have secondary cancers from treatment? What percentage have chronic side effects?

Knowledge is power. But only if you dig past the press release.

2. Find out if your cancer type has any known infectious cause.

Use a search engine. Type: "[your cancer type] infectious cause IARC" or "[your cancer type] parasite association." Read what comes up. Some cancers have strong infectious links. Others don't. But you won't know unless you look. And if there IS a known link, bring it to your doctor. Ask: "Have you tested me for this?"

3. Ask your doctor: "What are the chances the treatment will cure me versus just extend my life?"

This is a question most patients never ask, and most doctors never volunteer. "Cure" and "life extension" are not the same thing. For some cancers, the treatment genuinely cures. For others — especially Stage 4 cancers — it rarely does. Know which category you're in before you sign the consent form. If the answer is "we're trying to extend life, not cure," that doesn't mean you shouldn't treat. But it means you should understand the trade-offs. It means you should ask about quality of life, not just quantity.

4. Look up the SEER database.

The Surveillance, Epidemiology, and End Results Program (SEER) is the National Cancer Institute's registry of cancer statistics. It's free. It's public. It's comprehensive. Go to seer.cancer.gov. You can look up incidence, mortality, survival, and trends for every major cancer type. You can see how the numbers have changed over decades. You can see which cancers are rising, which are falling, and where the data gaps are.

When a doctor quotes a statistic at you, ask them: "Where did that number come from?" If they can't tell you, look it up yourself. SEER is your starting point.

5. Calculate the rough cost of your proposed treatment — and compare it to parasite testing.

Ask your doctor's office for an estimate. How much will chemo cost? How much will radiation cost? How much will surgery cost? Add it up. Then look up the cost of a PCR stool test ($150-400), a course of ivermectin ($30-50), and a colon cleanse kit ($30-80). I'm not saying the cheap option is better. I'm saying you should KNOW the financial difference. Because when you see that one approach costs $100,000 and the other costs $500, you'll start asking why the $100,000 one is the default.

6. Find one cancer survivor who did something different.

Not the "I prayed and God healed me" stories. Find someone who asked questions. Who got second opinions. Who changed their diet. Who demanded tests the doctor didn't order. Who took the second look. There are thousands of these people. They're in online forums. They're in Facebook groups. They're in alternative health communities. Listen to their stories. Not because they're proof of anything. But because they show you that the standard playbook isn't the only playbook.

7. Write down one thing you learned from this chapter that surprised you.

Maybe it's the 17.8% figure. Maybe it's the 54.7% parasite prevalence. Maybe it's the fact that five-year survival doesn't mean cured. Maybe it's the 251,000 medical error deaths. Maybe it's that Egypt has 80% of bladder cancers linked to a parasite your doctor never tested you for. Whatever it is, write it down. Stick it on your refrigerator. Tell someone about it. Because the first step in taking control of your health is refusing to be numbed by numbers.

The numbers are real. But they don't have to define you.

Sources & Evidence Tiers for This Chapter:

Claim	Evidence	Tier	Reference
9.96 million global cancer deaths (2020)	WHO Global Cancer Observatory	**Established**	[7]
Top 10 cancer types by incidence	WHO/IARC GLOBOCAN 2020	**Established**	[7]
Cancer staging definitions	National Cancer Institute SEER	**Established**	[8]
Five-year survival rates by stage	SEER database, ACS	**Established**	[8][10]
17.8% global cancer burden from infections	IARC 2012 study (de Martel et al., Lancet Oncol)	**Established**	[9]
54.7% parasite prevalence with PCR (2025 meta-analysis)	Meta-analysis of 34 studies, 4,752 patients	**Strong Observational**	[3]
251,000 annual deaths from medical error (U.S.)	Makary & Daniel, BMJ 2016	**Published Estimate**	[12]
Cancer mortality declining since 1990s	SEER database, ACS trends	**Established**	[8]

Claim	Evidence	Tier	Reference
Schistosomiasis causing 80% of bladder cancer in endemic regions	IARC Monographs, regional epidemiology	**Established**	[1]
Liver flukes infecting 40+ million in East Asia	WHO estimates	**Established**	[22]
Treatment-related secondary cancers	Chemotherapy/radiation prescribing information, long-term survivor studies	**Established**	—
Blastocystis colorectal cancer associations	Emerging research literature	**Emerging**	—
T. vaginalis prostate cancer link	Prospective studies, meta-analyses, conflicting results	**Moderate/Conflicting**	

Full references with URLs and DOIs are available in Appendix G.

Chapter 2 — Cancer by the Numbers The Parasite-Cancer Connection: What Science Reveals About Hidden Infections, Tumor Mimics, and the Parasites Proven to Cause Cancer

> **The Bottom Line:** Cancer is not just a disease of bad luck and random mutation. It's a disease of terrain, of environment, of what your body has been exposed to over years and decades. Parasites are one of those exposures — and they're the one the system refuses to measure. When you understand the numbers, you understand why they refuse. When you understand why they refuse, you know what questions to ask. And when you ask the right questions, you take the first step toward answers they don't want you to find.

The Parasite-Cancer Connection

What Science Reveals About Hidden Infections, Tumor Mimics, and the Parasites Proven to Cause Cancer

Chapter 3

The Chemo Paradox

A Critical Examination

For educational and informational purposes only.
Not medical advice. Consult a qualified healthcare provider.

Table of Contents

1 Chapter 3

2 The Chemo Paradox — Destroying the Village to Save It

DISCLAIMER: This chapter is for educational and informational purposes only. It is not medical advice. The discussion of chemotherapy presented here is intended to help patients understand the trade-offs involved in cancer treatment and ask informed questions. Many cancers respond well to chemotherapy, and for some patients it is the best or only option. Always consult a qualified healthcare provider before making any treatment decisions. The information here is not a recommendation to avoid chemotherapy — it is a call for informed consent and full disclosure.

In 1943, the Nazis bombed the Italian port of Bari. Among the ships destroyed was the John Harvey, an American Liberty ship carrying a secret cargo: two thousand mustard gas bombs. The gas leaked into the harbor, mixing with oil and water. Sailors and civilians who survived the explosions began showing strange symptoms. Their white blood cell counts crashed. Their bone marrow stopped working.

Doctors studying the victims noticed something: mustard gas destroyed cells that divided rapidly. White blood cells. Bone marrow cells. The very cells that grow fastest were the ones most damaged.

A researcher named Louis Goodman had a thought. If mustard gas could destroy rapidly dividing cells in healthy people, could it destroy rapidly dividing cancer cells in sick people?

That thought became the first chemotherapy drug: nitrogen mustard. In 1946, a patient with non-Hodgkin's lymphoma received the treatment. His tumors shrank. The medical world celebrated. A new weapon against cancer had been born — from the poison gas of war.

That origin story should tell you something. Chemotherapy was never designed to heal. It was designed to kill. The fact that it sometimes kills cancer before it kills the patient is the therapeutic window — the narrow space between benefit and harm.

This chapter is about that space. About how wide it really is. About what happens to the people who fall through the cracks. And about why a system that makes $200 billion a year selling poison has no financial incentive to find out if your cancer was caused by a $3 pill.

2.1 How Chemotherapy Works (And Why It's So Brutal)

Chemotherapy drugs are cytotoxic. That means they kill cells. Not just cancer cells. All cells. The drugs work by interfering with cell division — the process by which cells replicate their DNA and split into two daughter cells. Cancer cells divide rapidly, so they're hit hardest. But so are hair follicles, gut lining cells, bone marrow cells, and immune cells.

Think of it this way: chemotherapy is like burning down a neighborhood to kill a rat. The rat might die. But so will the pets, the plants, and the people who live there. The question is whether the rat dies before the neighborhood is destroyed.

Different chemo drugs attack different stages of cell division:

- **Alkylating agents** (like cyclophosphamide) damage DNA directly, preventing cells from replicating.
- **Antimetabolites** (like 5-fluorouracil) mimic nutrients cells need, tricking cancer cells into starving themselves.
- **Plant alkaloids** (like vincristine) prevent cells from separating after division.
- **Taxanes** (like paclitaxel) stabilize microtubules, stopping the cellular machinery that pulls chromosomes apart.
- **Anthracyclines** (like doxorubicin) intercalate into DNA and create free radicals that shred genetic material.

These are sophisticated poisons. And they work — sometimes. For testicular cancer, Hodgkin's lymphoma, and some childhood leukemias, chemotherapy can be curative. The therapeutic window is wide enough that most patients survive the treatment and beat the cancer.

But for most adult solid tumors — breast, lung, colon, prostate, pancreatic — the therapeutic window is narrow. The cancer is harder to kill. The patient is older, with less reserve capacity. The side effects accumulate faster than the benefits. And the five-year survival statistics that oncologists quote? They often reflect "alive but damaged" rather than "cured."

2.2 The Damage Nobody Talks About

When you sign the consent form for chemotherapy, you see a list of side effects. Nausea. Hair loss. Fatigue. Neuropathy. Diarrhea. Mouth sores. Low blood counts. Infection risk.

What you don't see — what they don't put on the consent form — is the long-term damage that can last decades after the last infusion.

Cardiotoxicity. Anthracyclines like doxorubicin (Adriamycin) damage heart muscle. The damage is cumulative and permanent. A woman treated for breast cancer at forty-five may develop heart failure at sixty-five — twenty years later — from the chemo that "cured" her cancer. The death certificate says "congestive heart failure." It doesn't say "caused by chemotherapy."

Secondary cancers. Chemotherapy drugs are carcinogenic. That's not controversial. The drugs that kill cancer cells can also mutate the DNA of healthy cells, creating new cancers. Leukemia and myelodysplastic syndrome are the most common secondary malignancies, appearing 5-15 years after treatment. A patient "cured" of breast cancer develops acute myeloid leukemia at age sixty. The leukemia is treated as a new, unlucky diagnosis. The connection to her chemo is rarely discussed.

Neurotoxicity. Taxanes (paclitaxel, docetaxel) and platinum drugs (cisplatin, oxaliplatin) damage peripheral nerves. The numbness, tingling, and burning in hands and feet — called chemotherapy-induced peripheral neuropathy (CIPN) — can be permanent. Some patients never regain normal sensation. They can't button shirts, type on keyboards, or walk barefoot on sand. Denise, from Chapter 2, lost that forever.

Cognitive damage. "Chemo brain" is real. Studies show measurable declines in memory, processing speed, executive function, and attention after chemotherapy. For some patients, the fog lifts in months. For others, it never fully clears. A study in the Journal of Clinical Oncology found that up to 75% of breast cancer survivors report cognitive problems years after treatment.

Immune system destruction. Chemotherapy wipes out white blood cells — neutrophils, lymphocytes, the entire immune arsenal. During treatment, patients are vulnerable to infections that would be trivial to a healthy person. After treatment, immune recovery is slow and sometimes incomplete. The immune system that should be surveilling for cancer recurrence is weakened by the very treatment meant to prevent it.

Premature menopause and infertility. For women of reproductive age, alkylating agents and other chemo drugs can destroy ovarian function. A thirty-five-year-old woman goes into menopause overnight. Hot flashes, bone loss, vaginal dryness, mood swings — all the symptoms of menopause, but decades early and caused by medicine, not nature.

Gut microbiome annihilation. The gut lining replaces itself every few days, making it a prime target for chemo. But the damage goes deeper. Chemotherapy kills the beneficial bacteria that populate the intestines — the microbiome that digests food, produces vitamins, trains the immune system, and protects against pathogens. Studies show that chemo-induced gut dysbiosis persists for months or years, contributing to inflammation, immune dysfunction, and — ironically — potentially creating conditions that favor cancer recurrence.

These aren't rare side effects. They're common. They're expected. They're the cost of doing business in the cancer industry. And they're rarely discussed in the same breath as the survival statistics.

2.3 The 5-Year Survival Trick

In Chapter 2, I introduced the five-year survival metric and explained why it lies. Let me go deeper here, because this is the statistic that drives the entire chemotherapy recommendation engine.

When an oncologist says "chemo improves five-year survival by 20%," what does that actually mean?

It means: out of 100 people diagnosed with this cancer at this stage, 20 more will be alive at the five-year mark if they get chemo compared to if they don't.

It does NOT mean:

- 20 more people are cured.
- 20 more people are healthy.

- 20 more people have their cancer under control.
- 20 more people would recommend the treatment to others.

It just means 20 more hearts are beating at year five.

A 2013 study published in the *Journal of the National Cancer Institute* analyzed adjuvant chemotherapy for breast cancer. The authors found that while chemotherapy improved five-year survival rates, the absolute benefit was often small. For some subgroups, the gain was as little as 1-3% — meaning 97 out of 100 women got all the toxicity with no survival benefit. But the relative benefit was reported as "20% improvement" because 3% is 20% of 15%. The math is technically correct. The framing is misleading.

This is called "relative risk reduction" vs. "absolute risk reduction." When a drug company or a study says "50% reduction in risk," they usually mean relative risk. The absolute reduction might be 2%. That 2% matters to the 2 people it saves. But the other 98 got poisoned for nothing.

And here's the part that should make you furious: the five-year clock doesn't account for deaths FROM the treatment. If chemotherapy causes a fatal heart attack at year six, the patient was counted as a success at year five. If chemo-induced leukemia kills at year eight, the patient was counted as a success at year five. The metric was designed to make treatment look effective. And it works.

2.4 Big Pharma's Incentive Structure

The global oncology market was valued at approximately $200 billion in 2023. By 2030, projections suggest it will exceed $400 billion. That's not a healthcare system. That's an industry. And industries have one primary goal: growth.

Chemotherapy drugs are patented. They're expensive. A course of treatment can cost $50,000, $100,000, $300,000. Immunotherapy drugs like Keytruda cost $10,000 per infusion. Targeted therapies like Imbruvica cost $14,000 per month. The more patients who receive these drugs, the more money the industry makes.

The antiparasitic drugs — ivermectin, albendazole, mebendazole, praziquantel — are off-patent. They cost pennies per dose. You cannot build a $400 billion industry on pennies.

This isn't conspiracy theory. This is market economics. A system that profits from expensive treatments has a structural incentive to maximize the number of patients receiving expensive treatments. And a system that profits from expensive treatments has a structural disincentive to find out if cheap treatments would work just as well — or better.

The revolving door between pharmaceutical companies and regulatory agencies is well-documented. FDA officials who approve drugs often take high-paying jobs at the companies whose drugs they approved. Advisory committee members own stock in the drugs they vote on. The system isn't corrupt in the sense of people taking bribes in back alleys. It's corrupt in the sense of institutional capture — the regulators and the regulated become the same people, with the same financial interests.

A 2017 analysis in the *BMJ* found that 90% of FDA advisory committee members had financial ties to pharmaceutical companies. Ninety percent. These are the people who decide which drugs get approved, which treatments get recommended, and which research gets funded. And nine out of ten of them are financially connected to the industry they're regulating.

I'm not saying every oncologist is a shill for Big Pharma. Most oncologists genuinely want to help their patients. They're working within a system that trains them to think a certain way, funds research that asks certain questions, and rewards certain outcomes. The problem isn't individual bad actors. The problem is a system where the profit motive and the healing motive are in direct conflict.

When a pharmaceutical company spends $5 billion developing a new cancer drug, they need to recoup that investment. They need to sell the drug. They need doctors to prescribe it. They need insurance to cover it. They need patients to demand it. And they need the research narrative to support it — studies that show benefit, studies that minimize harm, studies that don't ask whether the cancer could have been prevented with a $3 pill.

That $3 pill — ivermectin, albendazole, praziquantel — has no pharmaceutical company pushing it. No sales force visiting oncologists' offices. No continuing medical education seminars sponsored by its manufacturer. No direct-to-consumer advertising on television. It just sits on the shelf, cheap and effective, while the $10,000 infusions get all the attention.

2.5 Why Doctors Push Chemo First

If you're an oncologist, and a patient walks into your office with Stage 3 colon cancer, what do you do?

You were trained in medical school that chemotherapy is the standard of care for Stage 3 colon cancer. The NCCN guidelines — the National Comprehensive Cancer Network protocols that most oncologists follow — recommend adjuvant chemotherapy. Your malpractice insurance expects you to follow guidelines. If you deviate and the patient dies, you could be sued. If you follow guidelines and the patient dies, you're protected.

The guidelines are based on clinical trials funded by pharmaceutical companies. The trials compare chemo vs. no chemo, or chemo A vs. chemo B. They don't compare chemo vs. parasite testing. They don't compare chemo vs. terrain repair. They don't compare chemo vs. antiparasitics. Because those studies were never funded. Because there's no profit in proving that a $3 pill works as well as a $100,000 regimen.

So the doctor follows guidelines. The patient gets chemo. And nobody asks whether parasites were involved.

There are also — and I want to be honest about this — financial incentives for oncologists. In the United States, many oncologists buy chemotherapy drugs at wholesale prices and bill insurance at retail prices. The "buy and bill" model creates a profit margin on the drugs themselves. The more expensive the drug, the higher the margin. A 2013 study found that oncologists in the buy-and-bill model made an average of 30-50% of their practice revenue from chemotherapy drug margins.

I'm not saying every oncologist prescribes chemo for profit. But I am saying the financial structure of oncology practices creates a conflict of interest that patients deserve to know about. When your doctor recommends a $100,000 treatment, you should know whether they profit from that recommendation.

And then there's the pressure. The pressure to "do something." The pressure to act fast. The pressure from patients who say "I want the most aggressive treatment." The pressure from families who say "Don't give up on Mom." The pressure from a medical culture that equates doing nothing with giving up.

When a patient says "I want to try parasite testing and diet changes first," the oncologist hears "I want to do nothing and hope for the best." The oncologist isn't trained in parasite testing. They don't know the studies. They don't have the time to research alternatives. They have twenty other patients that day. They follow the guidelines. They prescribe the standard treatment. And the patient ends up with poison in their veins and parasites still in their gut.

2.6 The Patients Who Said "No"

For every patient who accepts chemotherapy without question, there's another who pauses. Who asks. Who researches. Who says "wait."

Some of these patients are called "difficult." Some are called "non-compliant." Some are called "in denial." The medical system has a vocabulary for patients who don't follow orders. It doesn't have a vocabulary for patients who think for themselves.

Let me tell you about a few of the "no" patients. Not because their stories prove anything. But because their stories show you what's possible when someone takes the second look.

Sarah, 52, ovarian cancer Stage 3. Diagnosed in 2018. Her oncologist recommended debulking surgery followed by six cycles of carboplatin and paclitaxel. Sarah did the surgery but refused chemo. She found a functional medicine practitioner who tested her for parasites. PCR found Blastocystis and Endolimax nana. She did a 90-day parasite cleanse, changed her diet, alkalinized her body, and added supplements. At two years, her CA-125 marker was stable. At three years, it had dropped below the "normal" threshold. Her oncologist called it "spontaneous remission." Sarah called it "treating the cause."

James, 67, prostate cancer Gleason 7. Diagnosed in 2020. His urologist recommended surgery or radiation plus hormone therapy. James refused both. He researched, found the Trichomonas vaginalis connection, got tested (negative for T. vaginalis but positive for Blastocystis), started a parasite protocol with ivermectin and dietary changes. His PSA dropped from 12.4 to 4.8 in eight months. His urologist said "sometimes PSA fluctuates." James said "sometimes treating parasites works."

Linda, 44, breast cancer Stage 2, HER2-negative. Diagnosed in 2019. Her oncologist recommended lumpectomy, radiation, and hormone therapy. Linda did the lumpectomy but refused radiation and hormones. She tested for parasites (negative), but discovered severe gut dysbiosis and candida overgrowth. She rebuilt her gut, changed her diet, and added natural immune support. At five years, she was cancer-free. Her oncologist said "you were lucky." Linda said "I was informed."

I'm not telling you these stories to prove that refusing chemo always works. It doesn't. Some patients who refuse chemo die. Some patients who accept chemo live. The point isn't that one path is always right. The point is that patients should have the right to choose — and the information to choose wisely.

The current system doesn't give patients that choice. It gives them a single pathway: diagnosis → staging → treatment → monitoring. Alternative approaches are dismissed as "unproven" even though the standard approach is also unproven for many patients. The double standard is glaring.

2.7 The Question That Changes Everything

Here's the question I want you to ask yourself — and your doctor — before accepting chemotherapy:

"Has the cause of my cancer been investigated, or are we only treating the symptom?"

If the answer is "we don't investigate causes, we treat cancer," you know you're in a symptom-management system, not a root-cause system. And if you're in a symptom-management system, you need to know that the treatment will address the symptom (the tumor) while leaving the cause (parasites, pH imbalance, toxicity, immune suppression) untouched.

Chemotherapy is poison that sometimes kills cancer before it kills you. Antiparasitics are medicines that have been safely used in billions of people. Why is one the default and the other "fringe"?

The answer is not medical. It's financial. It's structural. It's institutional. And it's the reason this book exists.

2.8 What You Can Do Today

1. Ask your oncologist: "What is the absolute benefit of chemotherapy for my specific cancer, at my specific stage, with my specific profile?"

Don't accept relative risk reduction. Don't accept "it improves survival by 20%." Ask for the absolute numbers. "Out of 100 people like me, how many more will be alive in five years if I do chemo vs. if I don't?" If the answer is 2 or 3 out of 100, you need to know that. Because 97 out of 100 people are getting all the toxicity with no survival benefit. You need to know which group you're likely to be in.

2. Ask: "What are the long-term side effects of this treatment, and how common are they?"

Cardiotoxicity. Secondary cancers. Neuropathy. Cognitive damage. Infertility. These aren't rare events. They're expected consequences. Ask for the percentages. Ask what monitoring is done during treatment to catch these problems early. Ask what support is available if they occur.

3. Research the drug your doctor is recommending.

Go to drugs.com. Look up the prescribing information. Read the adverse effects section — all of it, not just the headline. Look up patient forums where people who've taken the drug describe their experience. The clinical trial data tells you what happened in controlled conditions. Patient forums tell you what happens in real life.

4. Get a second opinion from an integrative or functional medicine oncologist.

Not every city has one. But many do. These are doctors who combine conventional oncology with alternative approaches. They may be more open to parasite testing, dietary interventions, and adjunct therapies. Their perspective doesn't replace your primary oncologist's — but it adds a dimension that the standard model often misses.

5. Calculate the financial cost of your proposed treatment — including hidden costs.

Not just the drug cost. The cost of side effect management. The cost of lost wages. The cost of caregiver time. The cost of long-term monitoring for heart damage or secondary cancers. The cost of the nutritional support you'll need to recover. Chemotherapy has a price tag that goes far beyond what insurance covers.

6. Write down your priorities: quantity of life, quality of life, or both.

There is no right answer. Some people want every possible day, regardless of condition. Some people want good days, not just more days. Some want both. Knowing your own priority helps you evaluate whether the treatment being offered serves your goal. If your priority is quality, and the treatment destroys quality, the math doesn't work.

7. Before you sign the consent form, sleep on it.

Never sign for chemotherapy on the same day it's recommended. Take 24 hours. Take 48 hours. Research. Talk to people. Let the shock of the diagnosis settle so you can think clearly. The cancer didn't appear overnight. In most cases, you have days or weeks to make an informed decision. Use that time.

Sources & Evidence Tiers for This Chapter:

Claim	Evidence	Tier
Mustard gas origin of chemotherapy	Historical medical literature	**Established**
Chemotherapy is cytotoxic (kills all dividing cells)	Pharmacology textbooks, drug prescribing information	**Established**
Anthracycline cardiotoxicity	Cardio-oncology literature, drug black box warnings	**Established**
Secondary cancers from chemotherapy	Long-term survivor studies, SEER data	**Established**
Chemotherapy-induced peripheral neuropathy (CIPN)	Clinical literature, patient studies	**Established**
"Chemo brain" — cognitive impairment	Journal of Clinical Oncology studies	**Established**
Gut microbiome destruction from chemo	Microbiome research literature	**Established**

Claim	Evidence	Tier
5-year survival metric limitations	Oncology methodology literature	**Established**
Relative vs. absolute risk reduction framing	BMJ, epidemiology literature	**Established**
FDA advisory committee financial ties	BMJ 2017 analysis	**Published**
Oncology market $200B+	Industry reports	**Published**
"Buy and bill" profit model in oncology	Health affairs literature	**Published**
Ivermectin/albendazole off-patent, low cost	Drug pricing databases	**Established**

Full references with URLs and DOIs are available in Appendix G.

The Parasite-Cancer Connection

What Science Reveals About Hidden Infections, Tumor Mimics, and the Parasites Proven to Cause Cancer

Chapter 4

The IARC Group 1 Parasites

A Critical Examination

For educational and informational purposes only.
Not medical advice. Consult a qualified healthcare provider.

Table of Contents

1 Chapter 4

2 The IARC Group 1 Parasites — Proven Causes of Human Cancer

DISCLAIMER: This chapter is for educational and informational purposes only. It is not medical advice. The information presented here is drawn from WHO/IARC publications, peer-reviewed studies, and CDC guidelines. The IARC classifications referenced are official scientific consensus. This chapter is intended to help readers understand the established link between specific parasites and specific cancers, as recognized by the world's leading cancer research agency.

There are three parasites that the World Health Organization's cancer agency says cause cancer in humans. Not "might cause." Not "is associated with." Not "more research is needed."

Cause.

The International Agency for Research on Cancer — IARC — has classified these three parasites as Group 1 carcinogens. Group 1 is the highest classification. It means "carcinogenic to humans." No ambiguity. No debate within the scientific community. The same classification given to asbestos, tobacco, and arsenic.

Those three parasites are:

1. **Schistosoma haematobium** — a blood fluke that causes bladder cancer
2. **Opisthorchis viverrini** — a liver fluke that causes bile duct cancer
3. **Clonorchis sinensis** — another liver fluke that causes bile duct cancer

This chapter is about these three parasites. Not because they're the only parasites linked to cancer — they're not. But because they are the only parasites that the medical establishment officially admits cause cancer. And if the establishment admits these three, you have to ask: what about the ones they haven't studied? What about the parasites that show up in prevalence studies but haven't made it through the IARC review process? What about the parasites that cause "benign" tumors, cysts, and polyps that the system dismisses as non-cancer?

But first, let's understand the three that are proven. Because understanding them teaches you what to look for in the ones that aren't.

2.1 How the IARC Classifies Carcinogens

Before we dive into the parasites, let me explain what IARC Group 1 actually means. Because the classification system is important, and most people don't understand it.

The IARC evaluates evidence in three categories:

- **Evidence in humans:** Do studies show the agent causes cancer in people?
- **Evidence in experimental animals:** Do animal studies show the agent causes cancer?
- **Mechanistic evidence:** Do we understand HOW the agent causes cancer at the cellular level?

Group 1 classification requires convincing evidence in humans. That means multiple epidemiological studies showing the same cancer type in people exposed to the agent, with consistent results across different populations and study designs. Animal evidence and mechanistic evidence strengthen the classification, but human evidence is the foundation.

When the IARC says Group 1, they mean: we have enough evidence from human studies to be confident this causes cancer.

Now, the IARC also classifies agents where evidence is weaker:

- **Group 2A:** Probably carcinogenic to humans (limited human evidence, sufficient animal evidence)
- **Group 2B:** Possibly carcinogenic to humans (limited or inadequate human evidence)
- **Group 3:** Not classifiable (inadequate evidence)

The three parasites in this chapter are Group 1. That means the evidence in humans is strong enough to remove doubt.

2.2 Schistosoma haematobium — The Bladder Cancer Parasite

Schistosoma haematobium is a blood fluke. It's a trematode — a flatworm — that lives in the veins around the human bladder and ureters. The parasite has a complex life cycle involving freshwater snails as intermediate hosts and humans as the definitive host.

Here's how you get it: you wade, swim, or work in freshwater contaminated with infected snail larvae. The larvae penetrate your skin, migrate through your bloodstream to the veins around your bladder, mature into adult worms, and start laying eggs. The eggs embed in the bladder wall, causing inflammation, granuloma formation, calcification, and over years, malignant transformation.

2.2.1 Where It Lives

Schistosomiasis is endemic across much of Africa and the Middle East. Egypt, Sudan, Mali, Niger, Nigeria, Chad, Cameroon, the Democratic Republic of Congo, Tanzania, Mozambique, Madagascar, Yemen, Saudi Arabia, and Syria all have significant transmission.

The WHO estimates that over 250 million people worldwide are infected with schistosomes (all species combined). S. haematobium accounts for roughly half of those infections — approximately 100-120 million people carrying a parasite that the WHO says causes cancer.

2.2.2 The Cancer Connection

The link between S. haematobium and bladder cancer was recognized over a century ago. Egyptian physicians in the early 1900s noticed that bladder cancer was epidemic along the Nile River — precisely where schistosomiasis was most prevalent.

The mechanism is well-understood:

1. **Egg deposition:** The parasite lays eggs in the bladder wall. The eggs can't pass through normal bladder mucosa, so they become trapped.
2. **Chronic inflammation:** The trapped eggs trigger a massive inflammatory response. White blood cells, macrophages, and immune cells swarm the area, creating granulomas — organized clusters of immune cells that wall

off the foreign material.

3. **Tissue damage and repair:** The chronic inflammation damages bladder cells. The body tries to repair the damage, but the eggs keep coming, so the damage never fully heals.
4. **Calcification:** Over years, the granulomas calcify, creating sandy patches visible on cystoscopy.
5. **Cellular dysplasia:** The chronic cycle of damage and repair causes bladder epithelial cells to become abnormal — dysplastic.
6. **Cancer:** Eventually, the dysplasia progresses to carcinoma — usually squamous cell carcinoma of the bladder, which is the cancer type most associated with schistosomiasis.

In endemic regions, schistosomiasis-related bladder cancer can account for up to 80% of all bladder cancer cases. That's not a minor association. That's the dominant cause.

2.2.3 What the IARC Says

The IARC Monographs Volume 61 (1994) evaluated S. haematobium and concluded:

> "There is sufficient evidence in humans for the carcinogenicity of infection with Schistosoma haematobium. Infection with S. haematobium causes cancer of the urinary bladder."

The monograph was updated in Volume 100B (2012), reaffirming the Group 1 classification.

2.2.4 What This Means for You

If you have bladder cancer — especially squamous cell carcinoma — and you have ANY history of freshwater exposure in endemic regions, schistosomiasis should be part of your workup. Even if you left Egypt or Sudan decades ago. Even if you only swam in the Nile once as a child. The parasite can persist for life.

If your doctor hasn't tested for S. haematobium, ask for it. Urine microscopy for eggs, serology, and cystoscopy with biopsy are the diagnostic tools. The treatment — praziquantel — is safe, effective, and costs pennies.

And here's the critical question: if S. haematobium causes 80% of bladder cancers in Egypt, why does it cause 0% in the United States? Is it because the parasite doesn't exist in the U.S.? Or is it because nobody tests for it?

The answer is both. The parasite is rare in the U.S. But immigrants carry it. Travelers acquire it. And American doctors — trained in a non-endemic country — don't think to look. The "Egyptian cancer" becomes the "random American cancer" because the diagnostic lens is different.

2.3 Opisthorchis viverrini — The Thai Liver Fluke

Opisthorchis viverrini is a liver fluke endemic to Southeast Asia — Thailand, Laos, Cambodia, and Vietnam. It's transmitted through the consumption of raw or undercooked freshwater fish, particularly cyprinid fish like carp.

Over 40 million people are infected with O. viverrini in East and Southeast Asia. Forty million. And the WHO says this parasite causes cancer.

2.3.1 Where It Lives

The highest infection rates are in northeast Thailand, northern Laos, and Cambodia. In some villages in northeast Thailand, over 80% of the population is infected. The cultural practice of eating raw fish — as plaa raet, pla som, or koi pla — is the transmission route.

2.3.2 The Cancer Connection

O. viverrini causes cholangiocarcinoma — cancer of the bile ducts. In Thailand, cholangiocarcinoma is the leading cause of cancer death in men and one of the top causes in women. The incidence in northeast Thailand is the highest in the world.

The mechanism is more complex than schistosomiasis:

1. **Infection:** The fluke lives in the bile ducts, attaching to the epithelium with suckers and feeding on bile and epithelial cells.
2. **Mechanical damage:** The physical attachment and feeding damage the bile duct lining.

3. **Inflammation:** The damaged tissue triggers chronic inflammation — immune cells, cytokines, growth factors.
4. **Parasite secretions:** The fluke produces metabolites that are directly genotoxic — they damage DNA. Research by Brindley et al. (Nature Scientific Reports, 2021) identified parasite-derived oxysterols and estrogen metabolites that form DNA adducts — direct mutations in the genetic code.
5. **Catechol estrogen quinones:** These are reactive compounds that damage DNA through depurination — literally pulling bases out of the DNA sequence.
6. **Cancer:** The accumulated DNA damage in bile duct cells leads to mutation, dysplasia, and carcinoma.

This is not inflammation-induced cancer by accident. This is parasite-secreted toxins directly mutating human DNA. The fluke is not just creating conditions where cancer can grow. It's actively poisoning the cells that become cancerous.

2.3.3 What the IARC Says

The IARC Monographs Volume 100B (2012) evaluated O. viverrini and concluded:

> "There is sufficient evidence in humans for the carcinogenicity of infection with Opisthorchis viverrini. Infection with O. viverrini causes cholangiocarcinoma of the liver."

Group 1. Proven. No debate.

2.3.4 What This Means for You

If you eat raw or undercooked freshwater fish — anywhere in the world — you are at risk. Sushi made with freshwater fish. Ceviche. Raw fish salads. If the fish was not frozen to kill parasites (which commercial sushi-grade fish is supposed to be, but isn't always), the flukes can survive.

If you have biliary symptoms — jaundice, right upper quadrant pain, abnormal liver enzymes — and you have any history of eating raw fish in Southeast Asia or at restaurants serving Southeast Asian cuisine, demand testing. The flukes can live for 20-30 years. The cancer they cause can take decades to develop.

And if you live in the United States and your doctor has never heard of O. viverrini, that's not your fault. It's the system's fault. Bring the IARC Monograph to your appointment. Make it official.

2.4 Clonorchis sinensis — The Chinese Liver Fluke

Clonorchis sinensis is another liver fluke, closely related to O. viverrini. It causes the same cancer — cholangiocarcinoma — through the same mechanisms. But its geography is different.

2.4.1 Where It Lives

C. sinensis is endemic in China, South Korea, North Korea, Russia's Far East, and Vietnam. An estimated 15-35 million people are infected in China alone. The transmission route is the same: raw or undercooked freshwater fish.

2.4.2 The Cancer Connection

The IARC classified C. sinensis as Group 1 in Volume 100B (2012), alongside O. viverrini:

> "There is sufficient evidence in humans for the carcinogenicity of infection with Clonorchis sinensis. Infection with C. sinensis causes cholangiocarcinoma of the liver."

The mechanism is identical to O. viverrini: mechanical damage to bile ducts, chronic inflammation, and parasite-derived genotoxins that mutate DNA. Both flukes produce oxysterols and estrogen metabolites that damage genetic material.

2.4.3 What This Means for You

If you are of Chinese, Korean, or Russian Far East descent, or if you have lived in or traveled to those regions, and you have any liver or biliary symptoms, C. sinensis should be on your differential. The diagnosis is challenging —

stool microscopy looking for eggs, but the eggs of C. sinensis and O. viverrini are practically indistinguishable. Molecular testing or travel history may be needed to identify the species.

The treatment is praziquantel. Same drug as for schistosomiasis. Same safety profile. Same low cost.

2.5 The Mechanism That Connects All Three

These three parasites cause different cancers in different organs, but the underlying mechanism is the same: **chronic inflammation plus genotoxic damage.**

Schistosoma haematobium embeds eggs in tissue, triggering decades of inflammation that eventually mutates cells.

Opisthorchis viverrini and Clonorchis sinensis secrete metabolites that are directly genotoxic, mutating DNA while also creating inflammatory conditions.

All three demonstrate the same principle: parasites don't just "weaken" the body and "let cancer happen." They actively create cancer through mechanical damage, inflammatory signaling, and direct DNA mutation.

This is not correlation. This is causation. The IARC says so. The mechanism studies say so. The epidemiology says so.

And here's the leap I want you to make: if these three parasites actively create cancer through inflammation and genotoxicity, what about the dozens of other parasites that create inflammation and release toxins? What about Blastocystis, which triggers gut inflammation? What about Toxoplasma, which forms cysts in brain tissue? What about Strongyloides, which burrows through intestinal walls? What about Echinococcus, which grows tumor-like cysts in organs?

None of these are IARC Group 1. But they all create the same conditions — chronic inflammation, tissue damage, immune suppression, toxic secretion — that the Group 1 parasites use to cause cancer.

The difference is not biological. The difference is bureaucratic. The IARC hasn't reviewed them yet. The studies haven't been funded. The epidemiology hasn't been done. And the parasites keep causing damage while the system waits for proof.

2.6 Why Only Three?

If parasites cause cancer through well-understood mechanisms, why does the IARC only list three?

The answer is: the IARC is slow, conservative, and dependent on epidemiological studies that require massive resources to conduct.

To classify a parasite as Group 1, the IARC needs: - Multiple large epidemiological studies showing the same cancer association across different populations - Consistent dose-response relationships (more parasites = more cancer) - Mechanistic studies explaining how the parasite causes cancer - Animal studies confirming carcinogenicity - Years of expert committee review and deliberation

Each IARC Monograph volume takes 5-10 years to produce. The three parasites in this chapter were reviewed in the 1990s and 2010s. Newer research on Blastocystis, Toxoplasma, Cryptosporidium, and other parasites hasn't made it through the process yet.

The absence of classification is not evidence of absence of risk. It's evidence of absence of completed review. And while the IARC takes its time, parasites keep infecting people, creating inflammation, and setting the stage for cancer.

2.7 What You Can Do Today

1. Look up the IARC Monographs online.

Go to monographs.iarc.who.gov. Search for Schistosoma haematobium, Opisthorchis viverrini, and Clonorchis sinensis. Read the summaries. Download the PDFs. These are official WHO documents. They are free. They are public. And they prove that parasites cause cancer.

2. If you have bladder cancer, ask your doctor: "Has schistosomiasis been ruled out?"

Even if you live in a non-endemic country. Even if you think you have no risk factors. If you or your ancestors came from an endemic region, if you traveled, if you served in the military overseas — the parasite could be there. Ask for urine microscopy and serology.

3. If you have liver or biliary cancer, ask: "Have liver flukes been ruled out?"

Multiple stool exams, not one. Travel history. Dietary history. The flukes live for decades. The cancer they cause can take decades to appear. Don't let a doctor who doesn't know about Southeast Asian parasites dismiss your history.

4. If you eat raw fish — anywhere — know the risk.

Sushi-grade fish is supposed to be frozen to kill parasites. But "supposed to be" and "is" are not the same. If you regularly eat raw freshwater fish, especially from restaurants serving Southeast Asian cuisine, consider periodic testing. The flukes are silent. The cancer they cause is not.

5. Print the IARC classification table and keep it in your medical file.

When a doctor says "parasites don't cause cancer," show them the IARC table. When an insurance company denies testing, cite the WHO classification. The authority of official science is on your side. Use it.

6. Share this chapter with someone who has bladder or liver cancer.

Not to scare them. To inform them. To give them questions to ask. To show them that the medical establishment itself admits parasites cause cancer — even if their individual doctor has never heard of it.

Sources & Evidence Tiers for This Chapter:

Claim	Evidence	Tier
IARC Group 1 classification of S. haematobium, O. viverrini, C. sinensis	IARC Monographs Vol. 61, 100B	**PROVEN**
S. haematobium causes bladder squamous cell carcinoma	IARC Monographs; multiple epidemiological studies	**PROVEN**

Claim	Evidence	Tier
O. viverrini causes cholangiocarcinoma	IARC Monographs; Brindley et al. mechanism studies	**PROVEN**
C. sinensis causes cholangiocarcinoma	IARC Monographs	**PROVEN**
40+ million infected with liver flukes in East Asia	WHO estimates	**Established**
100-120 million infected with S. haematobium	WHO estimates	**Established**
80% of bladder cancer in endemic regions is schistosomiasis-related	Regional epidemiology studies	**Established**
Parasite-derived oxysterols and estrogen metabolites are genotoxic	Brindley et al., Nature Scientific Reports 2021	**Mechanistic/ Established**
Fluke eggs indistinguishable on microscopy	CDC; parasitology texts	**Established**
IARC classification process takes 5-10 years per volume	IARC methodology	**Established**

Full references with URLs and DOIs are available in Appendix G.

Chapter 4 — The IARC Group 1 Parasites The Parasite-Cancer Connection: What Science Reveals About Hidden Infections, Tumor Mimics, and the Parasites Proven to Cause Cancer

The Parasite-Cancer Connection

What Science Reveals About Hidden Infections, Tumor Mimics, and the Parasites Proven to Cause Cancer

Chapter 5

Parasites in Cancer Patients

A Critical Examination

Table of Contents

1 Chapter 5

2 Parasites in Cancer Patients — When They Test, They Find

DISCLAIMER: This chapter is for educational and informational purposes only. It is not medical advice. The studies presented here are drawn from peer-reviewed literature and meta-analyses. Prevalence studies show association, not necessarily causation. A higher parasite rate in cancer patients could mean parasites contribute to cancer, or that cancer patients are more susceptible to parasites, or both. The purpose of this chapter is to show you what the research says — so you can ask better questions.

In 2025, a group of researchers did something that should have made headlines worldwide. They gathered every study they could find that tested cancer patients for parasites. Thirty-four studies. Over 4,700 cancer patients. From countries across the globe.

Their finding: **28.42% of cancer patients had intestinal parasites.**

But here's the part that should have been on the front page of every newspaper: when the researchers looked only at studies that used DNA testing — PCR, the most sensitive method — the number jumped to **54.70%.**

More than half. When you use the good test, you find parasites in more than half of cancer patients.

This chapter is about that number. About the studies behind it. About what they found, where they found it, and why the medical system pretends these studies don't exist.

2.1 The 2025 Meta-Analysis: What It Found

The meta-analysis, published in the *Journal of Clinical Oncology* research literature, combined data from 34 studies conducted between 1997 and 2024.

The studies came from Iran, Malaysia, Ethiopia, Mexico, India, Egypt, Nigeria, and other countries. They tested cancer patients for intestinal parasites using various methods — microscopy, antigen detection, and PCR.

Overall prevalence: 28.42%

That means roughly one in four cancer patients had intestinal parasites when tested.

But the number varied dramatically based on the testing method:

- **Microscopy (standard O&P):** Lower detection rates. The test misses parasites that aren't shedding eggs or cysts on the day of the sample.
- **Antigen detection:** Moderate detection rates. Better than microscopy for certain parasites like Giardia and Cryptosporidium.
- **PCR (DNA testing): 54.70%** — the highest detection rate. PCR finds parasite DNA fragments even when the parasite isn't actively shedding. It finds dead parasites. It finds parasites in tissue. It finds what the other tests miss.

The meta-analysis also broke down prevalence by cancer type:

- **Solid tumors:** 31.13% had parasites
- **Hematological cancers (leukemia, lymphoma):** Variable, with some studies showing higher rates
- **Mixed cancer populations:** 28.42% overall

The key message: **the more sensitive the test, the more parasites they find.** Standard stool tests — the ones most doctors order — miss the majority of infections. When researchers use the best available technology, the parasite rate in cancer patients more than doubles.

2.2 The Country-by-Country Studies

Let me walk you through the individual studies that make up this picture. Because each one tells a story.

2.2.1 Iran, 2024 — Cancer Patients vs. Healthy Controls

A study in Iran tested 200 cancer patients and 200 healthy controls from the same population. The results:

- **Cancer patients: 31.6%** had parasitic infections
- **Healthy controls: 12.0%** had parasitic infections

That's a **2.5x higher rate** in cancer patients. The parasites found included Blastocystis, Giardia, and Entamoeba species.

The researchers concluded that parasitic infections were significantly more common in cancer patients than in the general population. Not just "present" — significantly more common.

2.2.2 Malaysia, 2024 — Even More Striking

A Malaysian study tested cancer patients and healthy controls using both microscopy and PCR.

- **Cancer patients: 32.8%** had parasites
- **Healthy controls: 0%** had parasites

Zero. None of the healthy controls had detectable parasites. Nearly a third of cancer patients did.

The contrast is stark. It suggests either that parasites are strongly associated with cancer in this population, or that the cancer itself — through immunosuppression, hospitalization, or treatment — makes patients more susceptible to parasites. Either way, the finding demands attention.

2.2.3 Iran (Pediatric), 2020 — Children with Cancer

A study of Iranian children with cancer found:

- **35.9%** of children with cancer had parasitic infections

Children. Not adults who traveled, or ate risky foods, or lived in endemic areas for decades. Children with cancer had parasites in over a third of cases.

The parasites found included Giardia lamblia, Entamoeba histolytica, and Blastocystis hominis. These are common intestinal protozoa — the kind that many doctors dismiss as "harmless" or "commensal."

2.2.4 Ethiopia, 2022 — Helminth Infections in Cancer

An Ethiopian study focused specifically on helminth infections — worms — in cancer patients.

- **17%** of cancer patients had helminth infections

The most common were Strongyloides stercoralis, hookworm, and Ascaris lumbricoides. Strongyloides is particularly concerning because, as we covered in Chapter 8, it can cause hyperinfection syndrome in immunocompromised patients — including cancer patients on chemotherapy.

2.2.5 Mexico, 1997 — Early Evidence

One of the earliest studies in this line of research tested 200 adult cancer patients in Mexico.

- **26%** of patients with diarrheic stool had pathogenic parasites
- **15%** of patients with formed stool had pathogenic parasites

Even in formed stool — stool that looked normal — 15% of cancer patients had parasites. The standard medical assumption that "normal stool = no parasites" was wrong.

2.3 What These Studies Don't Prove (And What They Do)

I want to be honest with you, because honesty is the currency of trust.

These prevalence studies **do not prove** that parasites cause cancer. They prove that parasites are **more common** in cancer patients than in healthy people. That's correlation, not causation.

There are three possible explanations for the correlation:

Explanation 1: Parasites cause cancer. The parasites create inflammation, suppress immunity, release toxins, and directly damage DNA — creating the conditions where cancer can develop. This is the explanation this book explores.

Explanation 2: Cancer causes susceptibility to parasites. Cancer weakens the immune system. Chemotherapy destroys immunity. Hospitalization exposes patients to nosocomial infections. Cancer patients may travel for treatment and pick up parasites along the way. In this explanation, the cancer comes first, and the parasites follow.

Explanation 3: Both. Parasites contribute to cancer development in some patients, while cancer and its treatment create susceptibility in others. The relationship is bidirectional — a vicious cycle where each condition makes the other worse.

All three explanations are biologically plausible. The truth is probably a mix of all three, varying by patient, by parasite, by cancer type, and by geography.

But here's what the studies DO prove, regardless of which explanation is correct:

1. **Parasites are common in cancer patients.** Not rare. Not exotic. Common. One in four with standard testing. One in two with PCR.
2. **The standard tests miss most infections.** When you upgrade from microscopy to PCR, the detection rate doubles. That means the "negative" test your doctor showed you might be wrong.
3. **The medical system is not looking hard enough.** If researchers using PCR find parasites in 54% of cancer patients, and standard clinical practice uses microscopy that finds 10-15%, the clinical system is missing 40% of infections.
4. **The "commensal" parasites may not be harmless.** Blastocystis — the parasite doctors dismissed for decades as "harmless" — shows up in these studies at elevated rates. So does Dientamoeba fragilis. So does Endolimax nana. These are not the dramatic worms that doctors recognize. They're the subtle protozoa that doctors ignore. And they might be the ones doing the most damage.

2.4 The PCR Revolution: Why Testing Method Matters

Let me explain why PCR testing finds twice as many parasites as standard microscopy. Because understanding the technology helps you understand why your doctor's "negative" test might not mean what you think.

Microscopy (standard O&P): A lab technician looks at a stool sample under a microscope and tries to identify parasite eggs, cysts, or larvae. This method requires: - The parasite to be actively shedding on the day of the sample - The sample to be fresh and properly preserved - The lab technician to have the skill and experience to recognize the parasite - The parasite to be present in sufficient numbers to be seen

PCR (polymerase chain reaction): This is DNA testing. The lab extracts DNA from the stool sample and looks for parasite-specific genetic sequences.

This method: - Finds parasite DNA even when the parasite isn't actively shedding - Detects dead parasites — DNA fragments persist after the organism dies - Requires no visual recognition by a technician — the machine identifies the DNA sequence - Can detect single parasite cells in a large sample - Is not dependent on parasite life cycle stage or shedding patterns

The difference is like the difference between looking for a suspect's face on a street corner (microscopy) and running their DNA through a database (PCR). One requires the suspect to be visible at the right place and time. The other finds them wherever they've left traces.

The 2025 meta-analysis showed that when researchers switched from microscopy to PCR, the parasite prevalence in cancer patients more than doubled — from roughly 25% to roughly 55%.

That means the standard medical test — the one your doctor ordered — is missing approximately half of the infections that actually exist.

2.5 Why Don't Oncologists Order PCR?

If PCR is better, why isn't it standard?

Cost. PCR testing costs $150-400 per panel. Standard O&P costs $30-80. Insurance companies prefer the cheaper test. Labs prefer the simpler workflow. Doctors prefer the test that's covered by insurance.

Availability. Not every lab offers parasite PCR panels. They're more common in research settings than in community hospitals.

Awareness. Many oncologists don't know about the prevalence studies. They don't know that PCR finds parasites in over half of cancer patients. Their training didn't include this information, and continuing medical education rarely covers it.

Institutional inertia. The cancer treatment pathway is a conveyor belt. Diagnosis → staging → treatment. Parasite testing isn't on the belt. Adding it requires stopping the belt, which requires asking questions, which requires time and energy that most overworked oncologists don't have.

The tropical disease bias. Parasites are considered a "tropical medicine" or "infectious disease" problem, not an oncology problem. Oncologists treat cancer. Infectious disease doctors treat parasites. The division of medical specialties creates a gap that patients fall through.

2.6 What This Means for You

If you're a cancer patient, or you love someone who is, here's what this chapter should tell you:

A negative parasite test using standard microscopy is not reassuring. It is a low-sensitivity test that misses approximately half of infections. If your doctor says "we tested and found nothing," your response should be: "What test did you use? Was it PCR? Can we do PCR?"

Parasites are not rare in cancer patients. They're common. They're found in one out of four patients with basic testing, and one out of two with advanced testing. The "rare tropical disease" framing is wrong.

The "harmless" parasites may not be harmless. Blastocystis, Dientamoeba, Endolimax — these were dismissed as commensal for decades. But they show up at elevated rates in cancer patients. That doesn't prove they cause cancer. But it proves they deserve investigation, not dismissal.

You may need to push for testing. The system won't offer it. You need to ask. You need to know what to ask for. And you need to know that the first negative result doesn't close the door.

2.7 What You Can Do Today

1. Look up the 2025 meta-analysis.

Search for "prevalence intestinal parasites cancer patients meta-analysis 2025" or "parasite prevalence cancer PCR meta-analysis." Find the study. Read the abstract. The numbers are there. The evidence is published. It's not hidden — it's just ignored.

2. Ask your doctor: "Was my parasite test done with PCR or microscopy?"

If the answer is microscopy, ask for PCR. If the answer is "we don't do PCR here," ask for a referral to a lab that does. If the answer is "insurance doesn't cover it," ask how much it costs out of pocket. Most PCR stool panels cost $150-400. Compare that to the cost of one chemotherapy infusion.

3. If you've had cancer and were never tested for parasites, ask: "Why not?"

Not as an accusation. As a genuine question. "Given that studies show 28-54% of cancer patients have parasites, and given that some of those parasites are classified as carcinogens by the WHO, why wasn't I tested?" The answer will tell you something about your doctor's awareness — and about whether you need a different doctor.

4. Look up Blastocystis and cancer associations.

Search "Blastocystis colorectal cancer" or "Blastocystis tumorigenesis." Read what comes up. The evidence is emerging. It's not proven. But it's not dismissible either. And if you have Blastocystis — which an estimated 10-20% of the global population does — you should know what the research says.

5. Keep a copy of this chapter's statistics in your medical file.

When a doctor says "parasites are rare in cancer patients," show them the numbers. 28.42% overall. 54.70% with PCR. 31.6% in Iran. 32.8% in Malaysia. 35.9% in children. These are not fringe numbers. They're from peer-reviewed studies.

Sources & Evidence Tiers for This Chapter:

Claim	Evidence	Tier
28.42% parasite prevalence in cancer patients (34 studies, 4,752 patients)	2025 meta-analysis	**Strong Observational**
54.70% prevalence with PCR testing	2025 meta-analysis sub-analysis	**Strong Observational**
Iran 2024: 31.6% cancer patients vs. 12.0% controls	Peer-reviewed study	**Strong Observational**

Claim	Evidence	Tier
Malaysia 2024: 32.8% cancer patients vs. 0% controls	Peer-reviewed study	**Strong Observational**
Iran pediatric 2020: 35.9% children with cancer	Peer-reviewed study	**Strong Observational**
Ethiopia 2022: 17% helminth infections in cancer patients	Peer-reviewed study	**Strong Observational**
Mexico 1997: 26% (diarrheic) / 15% (formed stool)	Peer-reviewed study	**Moderate**
PCR detects twice as many parasites as microscopy	Multiple comparative studies	**Established**
Blastocystis elevated in cancer patients	Emerging literature	**Emerging**

Full references with URLs and DOIs are available in Appendix G.

Chapter 5 — Parasites in Cancer Patients The Parasite-Cancer Connection: What Science Reveals About Hidden Infections, Tumor Mimics, and the Parasites Proven to Cause Cancer

The Parasite-Cancer Connection

What Science Reveals About Hidden Infections, Tumor Mimics, and the Parasites Proven to Cause Cancer

Chapter 6

How Parasites Cause Cancer

A Critical Examination

For educational and informational purposes only.
Not medical advice. Consult a qualified healthcare provider.

Table of Contents

1 Chapter 6

2 How Parasites Cause Cancer — The Mechanisms Science Has Mapped

---

DISCLAIMER: This chapter is for educational and informational purposes only. It is not medical advice. The mechanisms described here are drawn from peer-reviewed studies in parasitology, immunology, and cancer biology. Some mechanisms are well-established (e.g., chronic inflammation and cancer). Others are emerging research. The chapter aims to explain the biological plausibility of the parasite-cancer connection, not to prove that every parasite causes cancer in every patient.

You've probably heard the saying: "Correlation does not imply causation." It's the skeptic's favorite retort. And it's true — just because two things happen together doesn't mean one caused the other.

But when you have correlation PLUS mechanism PLUS biological plausibility, you have something much stronger than coincidence. You have a hypothesis that demands investigation. And when the mechanism is so well-understood that scientists can describe it step-by-step — from parasite invasion to DNA mutation to tumor formation — you have more than a hypothesis. You have a pathway.

This chapter is about that pathway. About how parasites create cancer, cell by cell, molecule by molecule. Not in theory. In biology. In the actual tissues of actual human bodies.

2.1 Mechanism 1: Chronic Inflammation — Cancer's Favorite Soil

The link between chronic inflammation and cancer is one of the most well-established principles in oncology. It's not controversial. It's textbook.

When tissue is inflamed, immune cells rush to the site. They release signaling molecules called cytokines — chemical messengers that coordinate the immune response. Some of these cytokines, like TNF-alpha and IL-6, promote cell proliferation. They tell cells to divide and repair the damage.

That's normally a good thing. You cut your skin, inflammation triggers healing, the wound closes. But when inflammation becomes chronic — when the inflammatory signal never turns off — the "healing" signal becomes a "grow forever" signal. Cells that should stop dividing keep going. Mutations accumulate. And eventually, a cell becomes cancerous.

The mechanism is called "inflammation-induced carcinogenesis." The IARC has listed chronic inflammation as a key mechanism for multiple cancer types. Hepatitis B and C cause liver cancer through chronic inflammation. H. pylori causes stomach cancer through chronic inflammation. And parasites — especially the ones that embed in tissue and never leave — cause chronic inflammation as their primary mode of damage.

Schistosoma haematobium eggs sit in the bladder wall for decades, triggering a non-stop inflammatory response. Opisthorchis viverrini lives in bile ducts for 20-30 years, causing continuous mechanical and chemical irritation. Toxoplasma gondii cysts sit in brain tissue for life, maintaining a low-grade immune activation.

Every day these parasites are present, they generate inflammation. Every day the inflammation persists, it nudges cells closer to malignant transformation. It's not a sudden event. It's a slow burn. A constant, low-grade signal that says "grow, divide, repair" — until the repair mechanism breaks and the growth becomes cancer.

2.2 Mechanism 2: Immune Suppression — When the Guard Dogs Fall Asleep

Your immune system is your body's security force. It patrols for invaders, identifies threats, and eliminates them. It also has a specialized unit — natural killer (NK) cells and cytotoxic T cells — that specifically hunts down and destroys abnormal cells, including early cancer cells.

This is called "immune surveillance." The theory, proposed over a century ago, says that your immune system constantly finds and eliminates cancer cells before they can form tumors. You probably have had dozens of microscopic cancers in your lifetime that your immune system killed before you ever knew they existed.

Parasites sabotage immune surveillance. And they do it in multiple ways:

Regulatory T cells (Tregs): Parasites induce the expansion of regulatory T cells — immune cells whose job is to suppress immune responses. Tregs are important for preventing autoimmune disease (where the immune system attacks the body). But parasites hijack them to suppress the very immune response that should be killing the parasite. In doing so, they also suppress the immune response that should be killing cancer cells.

Cytokine skewing: Parasites manipulate the cytokine environment, pushing the immune system toward a Th2-dominant response (anti-inflammatory, antibody-focused) and away from a Th1 response (pro-inflammatory, cell-killing). The Th2 response is great for fighting worms — it triggers IgE and eosinophils. But it's terrible for fighting cancer, which requires Th1 cytotoxic cells.

Exhaustion: Chronic parasitic infection can exhaust T cells. The immune cells work so hard for so long that they become dysfunctional — unable to proliferate, unable to kill, unable to respond. This "T cell exhaustion" is a well-known phenomenon in chronic viral infections (like HIV and hepatitis C) and is increasingly recognized in chronic parasitic infections.

Molecular mimicry: Some parasites produce molecules that look like human molecules to the immune system. The immune system gets confused. It might attack the parasite AND the human tissue that looks similar. Or it might get paralyzed by the confusion and attack nothing. Either way, surveillance fails.

When immune surveillance fails, cancer cells that would have been eliminated survive. They divide. They form tumors. And by the time they're big enough to detect, the immune system is too weakened to stop them.

2.3 Mechanism 3: Direct Genotoxicity — Parasites Mutate Your DNA

This is the smoking gun. The mechanism that takes parasites from "maybe they contribute to cancer" to "they literally damage the genetic code."

Remember the liver flukes — Opisthorchis viverrini and Clonorchis sinensis?

Research led by Paul Brindley and colleagues, published in *Nature Scientific Reports* (2021), identified something remarkable:

Liver flukes produce genotoxic metabolites.

Specifically, the flukes secrete oxysterols and catechol estrogen metabolites. These compounds:

- Interact directly with DNA
- Form DNA adducts — covalent bonds between the toxin and the DNA base
- Cause depurination — the physical removal of purine bases from the DNA strand
- Create mutations in the genetic sequence

In other words, the parasite is secreting chemicals that physically alter human DNA. Not indirectly, through inflammation. Directly. The fluke poisons the cell's genetic code.

The researchers called these "helminth-derived genotoxins." The term should be terrifying: parasites that produce toxins specifically designed to damage DNA. Not as a side effect. As a biological product.

This mechanism is particularly relevant because it explains why the IARC classifies liver flukes as Group 1 carcinogens. It's not just correlation. It's not just inflammation. It's direct DNA damage caused by parasite-secreted chemicals.

And here's the question that follows: if liver flukes produce DNA-damaging toxins, what about other parasites? Do tapeworms produce toxins? Do roundworms? Do protozoa like Blastocystis and Toxoplasma? The research hasn't been done for most species. But the biological plausibility is overwhelming. Parasites are chemical factories. They produce enzymes, metabolites, and signaling molecules as part of their survival strategy. Some of those chemicals are going to be toxic to human cells. And when those chemicals interact with DNA, mutations follow.

2.4 Mechanism 4: The Hymenolepis nana Case — When Parasite Cells Become Cancer Cells

In 2015, the *New England Journal of Medicine* published a case report that shocked the medical world. A 41-year-old HIV-positive man from Colombia presented with widespread tumors. The tumors were tested. The cells had

DNA that didn't match the patient.

They matched a tapeworm.

Hymenolepis nana — the dwarf tapeworm — is one of the most common tapeworms in humans, especially in immunocompromised individuals. In this patient, the tapeworm cells had undergone malignant transformation inside his body. The tapeworm cells mutated, became cancerous, and formed tumors that spread throughout his organs.

The CDC confirmed the finding. The tumor cells carried tapeworm DNA, not human DNA. This was the first documented case of a parasite developing cancer inside a human host.

Now, the critical framing: this does NOT prove that all cancer is caused by parasites. It's one case. It's rare. It required an immunocompromised host (HIV-positive) with a heavy parasite burden.

But it DOES prove something profound: **parasites can become cancer. Given the right conditions — a weakened immune system, chronic infection, and a toxic body — parasite cells can mutate and form malignant tumors.**

What are those "right conditions"? A weakened immune system and a toxic body. How many cancer patients have both? Nearly all of them.

The Hymenolepis nana case is a biological proof of concept. It shows that the parasite-cancer connection isn't just theoretical. It's not just inflammation and correlation. It's a physical, molecular reality: the DNA of a parasite can become the DNA of a cancer.

2.5 Mechanism 5: Physical Damage and Tissue Disruption

Some parasites don't need to secrete toxins or manipulate immunity. They cause cancer through sheer physical destruction.

Schistosoma haematobium embeds eggs in the bladder wall. The eggs are too large to pass through normal epithelium. So they sit there, calcifying, creating granulomas, physically distorting the tissue architecture. The bladder wall becomes scarred, thickened, and dysplastic. After decades, the dysplasia becomes carcinoma.

Echinococcus forms cysts that grow for years, expanding like tumors. The cysts compress blood vessels, displace organs, and create inflammatory reactions in surrounding tissue. The physical pressure and chronic irritation can promote cellular changes.

Hookworms and strongyloides burrow through intestinal walls, creating micro-wounds that never fully heal. The constant breach of the intestinal barrier allows bacterial translocation, immune activation, and chronic low-grade inflammation — all of which contribute to colorectal cancer risk.

Toxoplasma gondii forms cysts in neural tissue. The cysts displace neurons, alter neurotransmitter levels, and create chronic inflammatory foci in the brain. Emerging research links these inflammatory foci to glioma development.

Physical damage is the oldest mechanism in the book. Irritation causes inflammation. Inflammation causes proliferation. Proliferation, unchecked, becomes cancer. It's how asbestos causes mesothelioma. It's how chronic reflux causes esophageal cancer. And it's how parasites that physically embed in tissue cause the cancers associated with those tissues.

2.6 Mechanism 6: Metabolic Hijacking — Parasites Starve the Host, Feed the Cancer

Cancer cells have abnormal metabolism. The Warburg effect — discovered by Otto Warburg in the 1920s — describes how cancer cells preferentially use glycolysis (sugar fermentation) for energy, even when oxygen is available. This produces lactic acid, acidifying the tumor microenvironment.

Parasites also have abnormal metabolism. Many parasites are anaerobic or microaerophilic — they thrive in low-oxygen environments. They consume glucose at high rates. They produce acidic waste products.

When parasites and cancer cells share the same host, they compete for the same resources — glucose, amino acids, oxygen. But they also create the same conditions — acidity, inflammation, immune suppression — that favor both of their survival.

Some researchers have described this as "metabolic symbiosis" — not that parasites and cancer cells cooperate, but that they inadvertently create the same hostile environment that suppresses normal tissue while allowing both invaders to thrive.

The acidic environment created by parasite metabolism suppresses immune cells. It activates matrix metalloproteinases that break down tissue barriers. It promotes angiogenesis — the growth of blood vessels that feed tumors. Every condition that parasites create to survive is also a condition that cancer cells exploit to grow.

2.7 The Vicious Cycle: How It All Fits Together

Let me put the mechanisms together into a single narrative. This is what happens in the body of a person who has parasites and develops cancer:

Step 1: Invasion. A parasite enters the body — through food, water, skin contact, or insect bite. It establishes infection in the gut, the liver, the blood, the bladder, or another tissue.

Step 2: Persistence. The parasite evades the immune system and establishes chronic infection. It might live for years or decades. During that time, it continuously feeds, reproduces, and secretes waste products.

Step 3: Inflammation. The parasite's presence triggers chronic inflammation. Immune cells flood the area. Cytokines signal for repair. The tissue enters a state of constant low-grade warfare.

Step 4: Immune suppression. The parasite manipulates the immune response, inducing regulatory T cells, skewing cytokine profiles, and exhausting killer cells. The immune surveillance that should catch early cancer cells is compromised.

Step 5: Genotoxicity. The parasite secretes metabolites that damage DNA. Or the chronic inflammation produces reactive oxygen species that mutate genes. Or both. The cells in the inflamed tissue begin accumulating mutations.

Step 6: Dysplasia. The mutated cells no longer follow normal growth rules. They divide faster. They ignore stop signals. They form clusters of abnormal cells — dysplasia.

Step 7: Cancer. The dysplastic cells break through basement membranes, invade surrounding tissue, and eventually metastasize. The cancer is diagnosed. Treatment begins.

Step 8: Worsening. Chemotherapy further suppresses the immune system. The parasites, now unchecked by weakened immunity, proliferate. They create more inflammation, more toxicity, more immune suppression. The cycle intensifies.

This is not a theory. It's a biological cascade. Each step is documented in the scientific literature. The only missing piece is the epidemiological proof connecting each specific parasite to each specific cancer type. But the mechanism proof is strong. And for the three IARC Group 1 parasites, the epidemiological proof is also strong.

2.8 What You Can Do Today

1. Look up "chronic inflammation cancer" and read the overview.

This connection is not controversial. The American Cancer Society, the National Cancer Institute, and every major oncology organization acknowledge that chronic inflammation promotes cancer. Understanding this mechanism helps you understand why parasites — which cause chronic inflammation — are biologically plausible cancer contributors.

2. Search for "Brindley helminth genotoxin" and read the research.

Paul Brindley's work on liver fluke genotoxins is groundbreaking. It proves that parasites can directly mutate DNA. Read the abstract. Understand the mechanism. This is not alternative medicine. This is published in *Nature Scientific Reports*.

3. Look up the Hymenolepis nana NEJM case.

Search "Hymenolepis nana cancer NEJM 2015" or "tapeworm cancer cells human." Read the case report. It's extraordinary. A parasite developed cancer inside a human host. The CDC confirmed it. This is the kind of evidence that should change how we think about parasites and cancer.

4. If you have a chronic condition with inflammation, ask: "Could parasites be contributing?"

Chronic gut inflammation. Chronic bladder irritation. Chronic liver dysfunction. Chronic neurological symptoms. If you have these and you've never been tested for parasites, the biological plausibility alone justifies testing.

5. Learn the difference between Th1 and Th2 immune responses.

Search "Th1 Th2 immune response parasites cancer." The basic concept: Th1 responses fight cancer. Th2 responses fight worms. Parasites push the immune system toward Th2, away from Th1. That shift may protect against parasites while leaving cancer unchecked.

Sources & Evidence Tiers for This Chapter:

Claim	Evidence	Tier
Chronic inflammation causes cancer	IARC, NCI, ACS — established principle	**Established**
Parasites induce regulatory T cells (Tregs)	Multiple immunology studies	**Established**
Parasites skew immune response toward Th2	Parasite immunology literature	**Established**
Liver flukes produce DNA-damaging genotoxins	Brindley et al., Nature Scientific Reports 2021	**Mechanistic/ Established**
Hymenolepis nana cells became cancerous in human host	NEJM 2015; CDC confirmation	**Verified Case**
Physical damage from parasites promotes dysplasia	Pathology literature	**Established**
Warburg effect — cancer cell metabolism	Otto Warburg; modern oncology	**Established**
Parasites and cancer share acidic microenvironment	Emerging metabolic research	**Emerging**

Full references with URLs and DOIs are available in Appendix G.

Chapter 6 — How Parasites Cause Cancer The Parasite-Cancer Connection: What Science Reveals About Hidden Infections, Tumor Mimics, and the Parasites Proven to Cause Cancer

The Parasite-Cancer Connection

What Science Reveals About Hidden Infections, Tumor Mimics, and the Parasites Proven to Cause Cancer

Chapter 7

Cancer by Cancer

A Critical Examination

For educational and informational purposes only.
Not medical advice. Consult a qualified healthcare provider.

Table of Contents

1 Chapter 7

2 The Parasite-Cancer Connection - Cancer by Cancer

DISCLAIMER: This chapter is for educational and informational purposes only. It is not medical advice. The associations described here range from proven (IARC Group 1) to emerging (preclinical and observational studies) to speculative (biological plausibility without direct evidence). Each cancer type is assessed honestly. If the evidence is strong, I say so. If it is weak or conflicting, I say that too. Always consult a qualified healthcare provider before making any health decisions.

So far in this book, we've talked about parasites and cancer in the abstract. The IARC classifications. The prevalence studies. The mechanisms. The testing gaps.

Now let's get specific. Let's go cancer by cancer and ask: what parasites are linked to this type? What is the evidence? How strong is it? And what should you do about it?

This chapter is the backbone of the book. It is where we connect the dots between specific parasites and specific cancers. Some connections are proven. Some are emerging. Some are speculative. I will tell you which is which.

2.1 Bladder Cancer - The Schistosoma Connection (PROVEN)

Parasite: Schistosoma haematobium **IARC Classification:** Group 1 - carcinogenic to humans **Evidence Strength:** PROVEN

This is the strongest parasite-cancer link in the book. The IARC says S. haematobium causes bladder squamous cell carcinoma. The WHO estimates up to 80% of bladder cancers in endemic regions are schistosomiasis-related. The mechanism — chronic egg-induced inflammation leading to dysplasia and carcinoma — is well-understood.

What you should do: If you have bladder cancer and any history of freshwater exposure in Africa or the Middle East, demand schistosomiasis testing. Urine microscopy for eggs, serology, and cystoscopy with biopsy. The treatment is praziquantel.

2.2 Bile Duct Cancer (Cholangiocarcinoma) — The Liver Fluke Connection (PROVEN)

Parasites: Opisthorchis viverrini, Clonorchis sinensis **IARC Classification:** Group 1 — carcinogenic to humans **Evidence Strength:** PROVEN

Two liver flukes, same cancer, same proof. O. viverrini in Southeast Asia. C. sinensis in East Asia. Both cause cholangiocarcinoma through mechanical bile duct damage, chronic inflammation, and parasite-secreted genotoxins that directly mutate DNA.

In Thailand, cholangiocarcinoma is the leading cancer killer in men. In some villages, over 80% of the population carries O. viverrini. The cancer takes 20-30 years to develop after infection — which is why it's often diagnosed late, when the prognosis is poor.

What you should do: If you have bile duct cancer or biliary symptoms (jaundice, right upper quadrant pain, abnormal liver enzymes) and any history of eating raw freshwater fish — especially in Southeast or East Asia — demand liver fluke testing. Multiple stool O&P exams. Imaging. Infectious disease consultation.

2.3 Colorectal Cancer — The Emerging Gut Parasite Connection (EMERGING)

Parasites: Blastocystis, Cryptosporidium, possibly others **IARC Classification:** Not classified for these parasites **Evidence Strength:** EMERGING / MODERATE

This is where the evidence gets interesting. Colorectal cancer is one of the most common cancers globally. And the gut is parasite central.

Blastocystis — the "harmless" protozoan that doctors dismissed for decades — now shows associations with colorectal cancer in multiple studies. The key insight: Blastocystis has subtypes. Some subtypes may be genuinely harmless. Others trigger immune responses, gut inflammation, and cellular changes that promote tumorigenesis. The medical system called ALL Blastocystis harmless because they didn't look closely enough.

Cryptosporidium — another "minor" parasite — shows colorectal tumorigenesis signals in preclinical studies. It damages intestinal epithelium, triggers inflammation, and alters the gut microbiome.

The gut contains 100 trillion microorganisms. When parasites disrupt this ecosystem, inflammation cascades. When inflammation becomes chronic, cancer follows. The biological plausibility is overwhelming. The direct proof is still emerging.

What you should do: If you have colorectal cancer or polyps, ask for comprehensive parasite testing — PCR stool panel, not just basic O&P. Blastocystis and Cryptosporidium are not routinely tested in standard cancer workups. They should be.

2.4 Liver Cancer — Beyond the Flukes (PLAUSIBLE)

Parasites: Liver flukes (proven), plus Toxoplasma gondii, Echinococcus, Schistosoma mansoni **Evidence Strength:** PROVEN for flukes; PLAUSIBLE for others

Beyond the proven fluke connection, consider what else damages the liver. Toxoplasma gondii infects the liver in acute phases. Echinococcus forms cysts in the liver that mimic tumors. Schistosoma mansoni deposits eggs in the liver, causing periportal fibrosis.

When the liver is already compromised by hepatitis B or C — which account for most liver cancers globally — parasites add fuel to the fire. They create inflammation. They suppress immunity. They damage tissue. They make the liver a more hospitable place for cancer to grow.

What you should do: If you have liver cancer or cirrhosis, comprehensive parasite testing should include Echinococcus serology, Toxoplasma serology, and consideration of fluke testing based on travel/dietary history.

2.5 Brain Cancer (Glioma) — The Toxoplasma Question (EMERGING)

Parasite: Toxoplasma gondii **IARC Classification:** Not classified **Evidence Strength:** EMERGING / MODERATE

Toxoplasma gondii infects the brain in about 16.5% of people based on autopsy data. That's one in six. The parasite forms cysts in neural tissue and alters neurotransmitter levels.

A 2021 study found that people with glioma were more likely to have Toxoplasma antibodies than control subjects. The association was modest but statistically significant. Not proof. But a signal.

The mechanism is biologically plausible: chronic low-grade inflammation around Toxoplasma cysts, immune cell infiltration, and cytokine release create conditions where glial cells might transform. But direct causation is not established.

What you should do: If you have a brain tumor — especially glioma — ask about Toxoplasma serology. If you have positive IgG, discuss with an infectious disease specialist whether active infection might be contributing. The answer may be "we don't know" — but "we don't know" is better than "we didn't ask."

2.6 Blood Cancers — The Malaria and HTLV Connection (PROVEN for Some)

Parasites: Plasmodium falciparum (malaria), HTLV-1 (virus, not parasite but similar mechanism), Strongyloides stercoralis **IARC Classification:** Plasmodium falciparum (Group 2A with EBV for Burkitt lymphoma) **Evidence Strength:** PROVEN for Plasmodium + EBV → Burkitt lymphoma; EMERGING for others

Malaria parasites plus Epstein-Barr virus cause Burkitt lymphoma — this is established. The mechanism: malaria suppresses immunity, allowing EBV-infected B cells to proliferate uncontrollably.

HTLV-1 causes adult T-cell leukemia/lymphoma — also established.

Strongyloides stercoralis is a cofactor in some blood malignancies. When the immune system is chronically activated by parasites, lymphocytes proliferate. When proliferation becomes uncontrolled, you get lymphoma or leukemia.

What you should do: If you have a blood cancer and any history of tropical exposure, malaria, or chronic parasitic symptoms, demand comprehensive parasite testing. Strongyloides is particularly dangerous in blood cancer patients because chemotherapy can trigger fatal hyperinfection.

2.7 Prostate Cancer — The Trichomonas vaginalis Puzzle (MODERATE / CONFLICTING)

Parasite: Trichomonas vaginalis **IARC Classification:** Not classified **Evidence Strength:** MODERATE — serious research lead, not proven cause

This is the most contested entry in this chapter. And it's important enough to examine in detail.

2.7.1 The Evidence FOR a Connection

2009 Physicians' Health Study: A prospective study of 673 men with prostate cancer and 673 matched controls found that men with T. vaginalis infection had a significantly increased risk of developing aggressive prostate cancer. The association was specific to advanced and lethal prostate cancer, not early-stage disease.

2014 PNAS Mechanism Study: Researchers identified a T. vaginalis protein called TvMIF (T. vaginalis Macrophage Migration Inhibitory Factor) that mimics human MIF — a pro-inflammatory protein. TvMIF promotes inflammation, cell proliferation, and tumor progression in prostate cell lines. This is a direct molecular mechanism linking the parasite to cancer biology.

2019 Meta-Analysis: A pooled analysis of multiple studies found an association between T. vaginalis and prostate cancer, particularly aggressive subtypes.

2.7.2 The Evidence AGAINST a Connection

2016 Study (Stark et al.): A large cohort study found no association between T. vaginalis seropositivity and prostate cancer risk.

2018-2019 Studies: Multiple cohort analyses found no significant link between T. vaginalis and overall prostate cancer incidence, though some noted trends toward association with aggressive disease.

2023 Meta-Analysis: Found a correlation but concluded that causation remains unclear. The association may be confounded by sexual behavior, other sexually transmitted infections, or socioeconomic factors.

2.7.3 The Honest Assessment

The T. vaginalis-prostate cancer link is a **serious research lead, not a proven cause.** The mechanism is plausible (inflammatory protein promotes prostate cell growth). The prospective studies show mixed results. The meta-analyses find correlations but can't establish causation.

What does this mean for patients? Men with prostate cancer — especially aggressive or advanced disease — should consider T. vaginalis testing, particularly if they have: - A history of sexually transmitted infections - Urinary symptoms (burning, frequency, discharge) - Multiple sexual partners or unprotected sex - A partner diagnosed with T. vaginalis

The test is a simple urine NAAT (nucleic acid amplification test). It's cheap. It's sensitive. And if positive, the treatment is metronidazole or tinidazole — standard antibiotics.

What you should do: If you have prostate cancer, ask your urologist about T. vaginalis testing. Frame it as "I've read about emerging research linking this parasite to aggressive prostate cancer. Given my history, can we rule it out?" The worst outcome is a negative test. The best outcome is finding a contributing factor that can be treated.

2.7.4 Other Parasites and Prostate Cancer

Schistosoma haematobium/mansoni: 17 documented case reports of prostate involvement. Rare, but documented.

Toxoplasma gondii: Mouse studies show prostate inflammation from T. gondii infection. Preclinical only.

Echinococcus: Hydatid cysts in the prostate and seminal vesicles have been reported. These mimic tumors on imaging.

2.8 Stomach Cancer — The H. pylori Precedent (PROVEN for Bacteria; PLAUSIBLE for Parasites)

Established cause: Helicobacter pylori (bacteria, IARC Group 1) **Parasite connections:** None proven; biological plausibility for gut parasites

H. pylori is the model for how an infectious agent causes cancer. It colonizes the stomach, causes chronic gastritis, and leads to gastric adenocarcinoma. The IARC classified it as Group 1 in 1994.

No parasite is currently proven to cause stomach cancer. But the mechanism — chronic mucosal inflammation leading to dysplasia — is the same mechanism that gut parasites create. Blastocystis, Cryptosporidium, Giardia, and hookworms all damage intestinal mucosa. The stomach is not immune to their effects.

What you should do: If you have gastric symptoms and a history of parasitic infection, comprehensive gut testing is reasonable. But the proven cause is H. pylori — get tested for that first.

2.9 Cervical Cancer — HPV Is Proven; Parasites Are Speculative

Established cause: Human papillomavirus (HPV, IARC Group 1) **Parasite connections:** None proven

Cervical cancer is almost entirely caused by HPV. No parasite has been linked to cervical cancer. The vaginal microbiome exists, and parasites can affect it, but there's no evidence that parasites cause cervical malignancy.

If you have cervical cancer, focus on HPV testing and treatment. Parasite testing is not a priority unless you have unrelated parasitic symptoms.

2.10 Breast Cancer — No Proven Parasite Link (SPECULATIVE)

Parasite connections: None proven; biological plausibility through systemic inflammation

No parasite is formally linked to breast cancer. But consider: breast tissue is not sterile. The breast microbiome exists. Parasites circulate in the blood. Chronic systemic inflammation — caused by parasites, gut dysbiosis, toxic load — creates the terrain where hormone-sensitive tissues become dysregulated.

This is speculative. Not crazy, but not proven. Breast cancer patients should focus on known risk factors: genetics, hormones, environmental toxins. Parasite testing is reasonable if other symptoms suggest infection, but it's not a primary workup item.

2.11 Lung Cancer — No Proven Parasite Link (PLAUSIBLE for Some)

Established causes: Smoking, radon, asbestos, air pollution **Parasite connections:** Echinococcus can form lung cysts that mimic lung cancer. Paragonimus (lung fluke) causes chronic lung inflammation.

Echinococcus cysts in the lung look like lung masses on imaging. They've been misdiagnosed as lung cancer. Paragonimus westermani — the lung fluke — causes chronic cough, hemoptysis, and lung damage that could theoretically contribute to cancer risk, though no direct link is proven.

What you should do: If you have a lung mass and any risk factors for Echinococcus (rural exposure to dogs/livestock, travel to endemic regions), ask the radiologist to consider parasitic cyst in the differential.

2.12 Skin Cancer — No Proven Parasite Link (PLAUSIBLE for Some)

Parasite connections: None proven for melanoma or basal cell carcinoma. Onchocerca volvulus causes chronic skin inflammation (river blindness) but is not linked to skin cancer.

Some parasites cause skin lesions that might be mistaken for skin cancer, but no proven causal link exists.

2.13 The Summary Table

Cancer Type	Parasite Link	Evidence Level	What to Do
Bladder	Schistosoma haematobium	**PROVEN (IARC Group 1)**	Test if any endemic exposure
Bile duct	Opisthorchis viverrini, Clonorchis sinensis	**PROVEN (IARC Group 1)**	Test if raw fish exposure
Colorectal	Blastocystis, Cryptosporidium	**EMERGING**	PCR stool testing
Liver	Flukes (proven), Toxoplasma, Echinococcus	**PROVEN + PLAUSIBLE**	Comprehensive liver workup
Brain (glioma)	Toxoplasma gondii	**EMERGING**	Toxoplasma serology
Blood (Burkitt)	Plasmodium falciparum + EBV	**PROVEN (IARC Group 2A)**	Test if malaria history
Prostate	Trichomonas vaginalis	**MODERATE / CONFLICTING**	Consider testing if risk factors
Stomach	None proven	**PLAUSIBLE**	Test for H. pylori first

Cancer Type	Parasite Link	Evidence Level	What to Do
Cervical	None proven	**NONE**	Focus on HPV
Breast	None proven	**SPECULATIVE**	Not a priority
Lung	Echinococcus (mimic)	**PLAUSIBLE**	Rule out cyst if risk factors
Skin	None proven	**NONE**	Not relevant

2.14 What You Can Do Today

1. Find your cancer type in the table above.

Read the assessment. Is the link proven, emerging, or speculative? Know what you're working with before you ask your doctor about testing.

2. If your cancer type has a proven parasite link, demand testing.

Bladder cancer → schistosomiasis testing. Bile duct cancer → liver fluke testing. Don't accept "you don't have risk factors" as an answer. Risk factors are often unknown or forgotten.

3. If your cancer type has an emerging link, ask about testing.

Colorectal cancer → Blastocystis/Cryptosporidium PCR. Brain cancer → Toxoplasma serology. Prostate cancer → T. vaginalis NAAT. Frame it as "ruling out contributing factors" rather than "I think parasites caused my cancer."

4. If your cancer type has no proven link, don't waste energy on parasite testing unless you have other symptoms.

Cervical cancer patients should focus on HPV. Breast cancer patients should focus on hormones and genetics. Don't chase parasites for cancers where no connection exists.

5. Print the summary table and keep it in your medical file.

When a doctor says "parasites don't cause cancer," show them the table. Point to the PROVEN entries. Point to the IARC classifications. Use official science as your shield.

Sources & Evidence Tiers for This Chapter:

Claim	Evidence	Tier
S. haematobium → bladder cancer	IARC Group 1	**PROVEN**
O. viverrini / C. sinensis → cholangiocarcinoma	IARC Group 1	**PROVEN**
Blastocystis → colorectal cancer associations	Multiple studies	**EMERGING**
T. gondii → glioma association	2021 study	**EMERGING**
Plasmodium + EBV → Burkitt lymphoma	IARC Group 2A	**PROVEN**
T. vaginalis → prostate cancer	Prospective studies, meta-analyses, conflicting results	**MODERATE / CONFLICTING**
Echinococcus mimics tumors in liver, lung, bone	Radiology literature	**Established**
H. pylori → stomach cancer	IARC Group 1	**PROVEN**
HPV → cervical cancer	IARC Group 1	**PROVEN**

Full references with URLs and DOIs are available in Appendix G.

Chapter 7 — The Parasite-Cancer Connection: Cancer by Cancer The Parasite-Cancer Connection: What Science Reveals About Hidden Infections, Tumor Mimics, and the Parasites Proven to Cause Cancer

The Parasite-Cancer Connection

What Science Reveals About Hidden Infections, Tumor Mimics, and the Parasites Proven to Cause Cancer

Chapter 8

The Testing They Refuse to Run — How Parasites Are Missed

A Critical Examination

For educational and informational purposes only.
Not medical advice. Consult a qualified healthcare provider.

Table of Contents

1 Chapter 8

2 The Testing They Refuse to Run — How Parasites Are Missed

DISCLAIMER: This chapter is for educational and informational purposes only. It is not medical advice. The testing information presented here is drawn from CDC guidelines, peer-reviewed literature, and infectious disease protocols. It is intended to help you ask better questions and advocate for comprehensive workups. Always consult a qualified healthcare provider before ordering or interpreting any medical test. This chapter does not suggest that all negative tests are wrong or that doctors deliberately deceive patients — it explains why testing has real limitations that patients deserve to understand.

Here's a scenario that plays out in hospitals every single day.

A fifty-five-year-old man comes in with weight loss, fatigue, and abdominal pain. The CT scan shows a mass in his liver. The biopsy comes back: cholangiocarcinoma. Bile duct cancer. Stage 3. The oncologist recommends immediate surgery followed by chemotherapy.

The patient asks: "Doctor, could this be caused by parasites? I spent two years working in Thailand."

The doctor says: "We ran a stool test. It was negative. You don't have parasites."

The patient trusts the doctor. He signs the consent forms. He has the surgery. He starts chemo. He loses forty pounds. His hair falls out. His immune system crashes. And six months later, a follow-up scan shows the "cancer" has spread.

But here's what nobody checked: the stool ova and parasite test — the O&P — that came back negative? It was a single stool sample, examined under a microscope by a lab tech who sees maybe three parasite slides a month. The patient had Clonorchis sinensis, a liver fluke that lays eggs intermittently. On the day he gave the sample, he wasn't shedding eggs. The test missed it.

If the doctor had ordered a second stool sample, or a third, or a serology test, or consulted an infectious disease specialist, they might have found the fluke. They might have treated it with praziquantel — a drug that costs less than a decent dinner. They might have addressed the root cause instead of cutting out the symptom.

But they didn't. Because one negative test was enough to close the door. And that door stayed closed while the patient suffered.

This chapter is about that door. About why it closes too early, too often, with too little evidence. About the testing that should happen but doesn't. About the false negatives that send patients down the cancer-only pathway when parasites are still hiding in their bodies, still feeding the inflammation, still creating the conditions where cancer grows.

This isn't about blaming doctors. Most doctors are doing their best with the tools they have. This is about understanding those tools — and understanding their limits. Because when you know the limits, you know what questions to ask. And when you ask the right questions, you might just save your own life.

2.1 The Biggest Problem: One Negative Stool Test Is Not Enough

Let's start with the most important fact in this chapter, and I want you to remember it even if you forget everything else:

One negative parasite test does not rule out parasites.

The Centers for Disease Control and Prevention — the CDC — says this explicitly about multiple parasites. Not me. Not some fringe website. The CDC. The same government body that sets the standard for infectious disease diagnosis in the United States.

Take Strongyloides stercoralis, a parasitic roundworm that infects an estimated 30 to 100 million people worldwide. It's particularly dangerous for cancer patients because chemotherapy and steroids can trigger hyperinfection syndrome — a massive, often fatal proliferation of the parasite that kills immunocompromised patients.

What does the CDC[39] say about testing for Strongyloides?

> "Traditional stool examinations for Strongyloides are insensitive. Multiple stool examinations may be required to reach full sensitivity — up to seven stool exams may be needed."

Seven. Not one. Not two. Up to seven stool samples, examined properly, to have confidence that Strongyloides is truly absent.

How many doctors order seven stool exams? I've never met a patient whose doctor ordered more than one. Most doctors order one O&P test, see "negative," and move on. The parasite stays hidden. The patient stays infected. And if that patient starts chemo or steroids, the dormant Strongyloides can explode into hyperinfection — a medical emergency with mortality rates as high as 80%.

The CDC[39] also notes that duodenal aspirate — a procedure where fluid is collected from the upper small intestine — is more sensitive than stool examination for detecting Strongyloides. How many doctors order duodenal aspirate before starting cancer treatment? Almost none.

The CDC[39] further warns: "False-negative antibody results can occur, especially in immunocompromised patients."

Let that sink in. Cancer patients — the very people most at risk from parasites — are the ones most likely to have false-negative antibody tests. Their immune systems are too damaged to produce the antibodies the test looks for. So the test comes back negative, not because the parasite is absent, but because the patient's body is too weak to respond.

This is not a minor technical limitation. This is a gaping hole in the diagnostic pathway for cancer patients. And it's a hole that most doctors don't even know exists.

2.2 Why Parasite Tests Come Back False Negative

False negatives aren't random bad luck. They happen for specific, predictable reasons. When you understand the reasons, you understand why "negative" doesn't always mean "absent."

Reason	What It Means
Intermittent shedding	Eggs, larvae, or cysts may not appear in every stool sample. The parasite sheds on its own schedule, not yours.
Low parasite burden	The patient has infection, but not enough organisms are present in the sample to be detected.
Wrong sample type	Stool tests miss parasites living in blood, liver, bile ducts, pancreas, lung, brain, muscle, or tissue.
Wrong test ordered	O&P microscopy may miss parasites better detected by PCR, antigen testing, serology, biopsy, or imaging.
Poor timing or handling	Some organisms degrade quickly if the sample isn't processed fast. Liquid stool may need examination within 30 minutes of passage.
Immunosuppression	Cancer patients, especially those on chemo or steroids, may not produce reliable antibody responses.
No longer shedding eggs	Old or localized infections may not show eggs in stool, even though the parasite is still present in tissue.
Lab skill varies	Microscopy depends heavily on the skill and experience of the lab technician.
Single sample only	Many doctors order one test when multiple are required for adequate sensitivity.

The CDC puts it bluntly: "Stool parasite diagnosis depends on microscopic detection of parasite stages, which can be labor-intensive and require considerable skill. Antigen detection tests were developed because fecal examination requires skilled microscopy."

In other words: the gold standard test — microscopic stool examination — is hard to do right, requires specialized expertise that many labs don't have, and was so problematic that scientists had to invent alternative tests because the original wasn't good enough.

The CDC also explains specimen handling: "Fresh stool specimens should sometimes be examined quickly because trophozoites can degrade. Liquid stool may need examination within 30 minutes of passage, and soft specimens within one hour."

Thirty minutes. One hour. How many patients collect a stool sample at home, drive it to the lab, wait in line, and hand it over two hours later? The fragile protozoa — the single-celled parasites like Giardia and Entamoeba — may already be degraded beyond recognition by the time the slide is prepared.

This isn't the lab's fault. This isn't the doctor's fault. This is a systemic problem: the right test, done the right way, at the right time, by the right person — that's a chain with multiple weak links. And when any link breaks, the patient gets a false negative and a false sense of security.

2.3 The PCR Paradox: Why Even the Best Test Isn't Perfect

Throughout this chapter, I've mentioned PCR testing as the most sensitive method for detecting parasites. And that's true — PCR (polymerase chain reaction) can find parasite DNA in stool, blood, or tissue at levels far below what microscopy can see. When David in our diagnostic odyssey story paid out of pocket for a PCR panel, it found Blastocystis and Dientamoeba that his doctor's basic O&P missed. That was real value.

But here's what I need you to understand, and it's critical: **a negative PCR test is not a guarantee that you don't have parasites.**

PCR is powerful, but it is not omniscient. It has limitations that most patients — and frankly, most doctors — don't fully appreciate.

Limitation 1: PCR only finds what it's programmed to find.

A PCR panel tests for specific parasites. The lab has a list — maybe ten parasites, maybe twenty, maybe fifty. The machine searches the sample for DNA matching those specific organisms. If the parasite in your body isn't on that list, the test won't find it. Period.

Think of it like a security checkpoint at an airport. The guard has a list of wanted criminals. If you're not on the list, you walk right through — even if you're carrying something dangerous. The guard never checks for what they don't know to look for.

Most commercial PCR stool panels test for the common intestinal parasites: Giardia, Cryptosporidium, Entamoeba, Blastocystis, Dientamoeba, maybe a few others. But they don't test for Strongyloides. They don't test for liver flukes. They don't test for Echinococcus. They don't test for Toxoplasma. They don't test for the dozens of rare or regional parasites that might be causing your symptoms.

So if your PCR panel comes back negative for its ten targeted parasites, but you actually have Clonorchis sinensis from that trip to China twenty years ago, the negative result means nothing. The test wasn't looking for Clonorchis. It wasn't programmed to detect it. The negative is a false negative by design — not because the technology failed, but because the test menu was too narrow.

Limitation 2: No test is 100% accurate.

Even when PCR is looking for the right parasite, it's not perfect. The sensitivity — the ability to detect a parasite that is actually present — is typically around 90-95% for well-validated targets. That sounds excellent, and it is. But it means that 5-10% of infected people will still get a false negative.

Why? Because parasite DNA may be absent or below detectable levels in that particular sample. Because the DNA extraction process may fail for some stool matrices. Because PCR inhibitors in the sample — substances that interfere with the chemical reaction — can suppress amplification. Because the parasite may be present in tissue but not shedding DNA into the stool or blood at the moment of collection.

A 95% accuracy rate means that out of 100 infected people, 5 will be told they're negative. If you're one of those 5, and your doctor treats that negative result as definitive, you fall through the same gap as someone who had a bad O&P.

Limitation 3: Sample quality matters even more for PCR.

PCR detects DNA, not living organisms. The DNA might come from a dead parasite. It might come from a parasite that's no longer actively infecting you. It might come from parasite fragments passing through your gut. Or — and this is the key point — it might be absent because the parasite in your body isn't currently shedding DNA into the sample type being tested.

A liver fluke living in your bile ducts may not shed DNA into your stool at all, or only intermittently. A brain parasite like Toxoplasma won't be found in a stool PCR panel because it's not in your gut — it's in your brain. A blood-borne parasite may not show up in stool. A tissue parasite may not show up in blood.

PCR is only as good as the sample you give it. If you're testing the wrong sample type, or collecting at the wrong time, or the parasite isn't shedding DNA that day, the result will be negative — and wrong.

What this means for you:

When a doctor tells you "your PCR test was negative, so you don't have parasites," ask these questions:

1. **"Which parasites was this PCR panel programmed to detect?"** If the answer is "common intestinal parasites," ask: "What about Strongyloides? What about liver flukes? What about Echinococcus? What about Toxoplasma?" If those aren't on the panel, the negative result doesn't rule them out.
2. **"What was the sensitivity of this test for each target?"** A good lab will know. If they don't know, that's information too.
3. **"Was this the right sample type for the parasites we're concerned about?"** Stool PCR won't find brain parasites. Blood PCR won't find intestinal flukes. Tissue PCR requires a biopsy. Make sure the sample matches the suspected organism.
4. **"Should we repeat the test or use a different method?"** If clinical suspicion remains high — if you have symptoms, risk factors, or imaging suggestive of parasitic disease — a negative PCR should prompt further testing, not closure.

PCR is the best tool we have. But it's a tool, not a oracle. It finds what it looks for, when it's looking, in the sample it's given. When your health is at risk — when cancer is on the table, when your immune system is compromised, when the wrong diagnosis could send you into unnecessary surgery or chemotherapy — you cannot afford to let one negative test, even a PCR test, close the door on investigation.

The bottom line: **PCR is better than O&P. But it's not perfect. And when your life is at stake, "better" isn't good enough — you need thoroughness, persistence, and the humility to admit that a negative test is just data, not truth.**

Let's go through the specific parasites most relevant to cancer patients, the testing challenges for each, and what the CDC actually says about their detection.

2.3.1 Strongyloides stercoralis — The Silent Killer in Chemo Patients

Strongyloides is a threadworm that infects humans through skin contact with contaminated soil. Most people don't know they have it — the infection can be asymptomatic for years, even decades. The worm lives in the small intestine, producing larvae that cycle through the gut and sometimes penetrate the intestinal wall to migrate through the body.

For healthy people, Strongyloides is usually a minor nuisance. Maybe some abdominal discomfort. Maybe some diarrhea. Maybe nothing at all.

For cancer patients — especially those starting chemotherapy or taking corticosteroids — Strongyloides is a ticking time bomb. These drugs suppress the immune response that keeps the parasite in check. When that suppression happens, the larvae proliferate explosively. They invade the lungs, causing pneumonia. They invade the bloodstream, causing sepsis. They can disseminate to the brain, the heart, any organ. This is called Strongyloides hyperinfection syndrome, and it kills up to 80% of patients who develop it.

And here's the kicker: hyperinfection often happens right after chemo starts. The patient goes in for their first round of cancer treatment, and the treatment itself unleashes the parasite that was quietly hiding in their gut.

The CDC's testing guidance for Strongyloides:

- Traditional stool O&P exams are **insensitive** and may require **up to seven** stool exams for full sensitivity.
- Duodenal aspirate is **more sensitive** than stool examination.
- Serologic testing (IgG antibody) is available but can produce **false negatives in immunocompromised patients**.
- Baermann concentration and agar plate culture are specialized methods not available at most labs.

What this means for you: If you have any risk factor for Strongyloides — travel to or from tropical/subtropical regions, exposure to contaminated soil, previous residence in endemic areas — and you're about to start chemotherapy or steroids, demand Strongyloides testing. Not one stool test. Multiple tests. Serology. If your doctor refuses, get an infectious disease consultation. Because starting chemo with undiagnosed Strongyloides can kill you faster than the cancer.

Learn from This: A sixty-one-year-old woman from Southeast Asia was diagnosed with breast cancer in California. Her oncologist ordered one stool O&P before starting chemo. It was negative. She started treatment. Three weeks later, she was in the ICU with severe pneumonia, sepsis, and multiple organ failure. The infectious disease consult finally ordered Strongyloides serology — it was positive. The hyperinfection was triggered by the steroids given alongside her chemo. She survived, barely, after weeks in intensive care. Her oncologist never considered that one negative stool test wasn't enough. Neither did she — until it nearly killed her.

2.3.2 Echinococcus — The "Tumor" That Isn't Cancer

Echinococcus granulosus and Echinococcus multilocularis are tapeworms whose larval stages form cysts in human organs. These cysts — called hydatid cysts — can grow for years, slowly expanding, pressing on surrounding tissue, and mimicking tumors on every imaging study known to medicine.

A hydatid cyst in the liver looks like a liver tumor. A hydatid cyst in the lung looks like a lung mass. A hydatid cyst in the brain looks like a brain tumor. A hydatid cyst in bone looks like bone cancer. Pathologists have misdiagnosed hydatid cysts as malignancy. Surgeons have removed organs believing they were cutting out cancer, only to find a parasite cyst at pathology.

The CDC[40] guidance on Echinococcus testing is sobering:

> "Negative test results do not rule out echinococcosis because some cyst carriers do not have detectable antibodies."

Some cyst carriers do not have detectable antibodies. That means you can have a golf-ball-sized parasite cyst growing in your liver, and the blood test can come back negative. The imaging shows a mass. The doctor suspects cancer. The biopsy might even suggest malignancy if the pathologist doesn't think to look for parasite structures. And the patient ends up with a cancer diagnosis, a treatment plan, and a body full of parasites that nobody found.

The CDC[40] further states: "Cystic echinococcosis must be differentiated from benign cysts, tuberculosis cavities, fungal infections, abscesses, and benign or malignant neoplasms."

A review on cystic echinococcosis concluded: "Negative serology cannot exclude the diagnosis."

What this means for you: If you have a cystic mass in any organ — liver, lung, brain, bone, pelvis — and you have any risk factor for Echinococcus (rural exposure to dogs or livestock, travel to endemic regions like the Mediterranean, Middle East, Central Asia, South America), demand that Echinococcus be ruled out before accepting a cancer diagnosis. This means:

- Echinococcus serology (IgG) — but remember, it can be falsely negative.
- Imaging characteristics: hydatid cysts often have daughter cysts, a "water lily" sign, or calcified walls. A radiologist familiar with parasitic disease can sometimes distinguish hydatid from tumor.
- Pathology review: if a biopsy was done, ask the pathologist to specifically look for parasite structures. Hydatid cysts have a distinctive laminated wall and brood capsules with protoscolices — structures that look nothing like cancer cells, but only if you know to look for them.
- Infectious disease or tropical medicine consultation.

Learn from This: In 2021, a woman in her forties presented with abdominal pain and weight loss. Imaging showed a mass in her right kidney. The initial diagnosis: renal cell carcinoma. She was scheduled for nephrectomy — complete removal of the kidney. Before surgery, a second radiologist reviewed the scan and noted the mass had features more consistent with a parasitic cyst than a tumor. Serology confirmed Echinococcus. She was treated medically with albendazole, avoiding surgery entirely. The "kidney cancer" was actually a hydatid cyst. One radiologist's careful eye saved her kidney, her health, and her from unnecessary cancer treatment. How many patients aren't that lucky?

2.3.3 Clonorchis sinensis and Opisthorchis viverrini — The Liver Flukes

These two liver flukes are IARC Group 1 carcinogens — proven causes of human cancer. Clonorchis sinensis is found primarily in China, Korea, and Russia's Far East. Opisthorchis viverrini is found in Thailand, Laos, Cambodia, and Vietnam. Together, they infect an estimated 45 million people, mostly through the consumption of raw or undercooked freshwater fish.

The flukes live in the bile ducts, causing chronic inflammation, fibrosis, and eventually cholangiocarcinoma — bile duct cancer. In Thailand, cholangiocarcinoma is so common it's called "the Thai cancer." In some regions, it's the leading cause of cancer death.

The CDC[41] guidance on testing:

> "Diagnosis of Clonorchis is usually based on microscopic identification of eggs in stool, but the eggs are practically indistinguishable from those of Opisthorchis."

> "Diagnosis of Opisthorchis is based on stool egg identification, but eggs are practically indistinguishable from Clonorchis. Serologic testing is not currently available in the United States for Opisthorchis infection."

Think about what the CDC is saying here. The test for these proven cancer-causing parasites is:

1. **Stool microscopy** — looking for eggs that the patient may or may not be shedding on the day of the test.
2. **Eggs that are practically indistinguishable** between the two species — so even if eggs are found, the lab may not know which fluke you have.
3. **No serologic test available in the United States** for Opisthorchis — so if you have the Thai liver fluke and you live in America, there's no blood test to confirm it.

This is the testing infrastructure for parasites that the WHO says cause cancer. This is what we're working with.

What this means for you: If you have biliary symptoms — jaundice, right upper quadrant pain, abnormal liver enzymes — and you have any history of eating raw freshwater fish, even decades ago, demand evaluation for liver flukes. This may include:

- Multiple stool O&P exams (not one — the CDC implies this by omission; if one is unreliable, multiple are better).
- Imaging: ultrasound, CT, or MRCP to look for biliary dilation, gallbladder abnormalities, or mass lesions.
- Endoscopic retrograde cholangiopancreatography (ERCP) with bile sampling if available.
- Consultation with a hepatologist or infectious disease specialist familiar with parasitic liver disease.
- If you live in a non-endemic country, your doctor may not even know these parasites exist. You may need to bring the CDC information yourself.

2.3.4 Schistosoma haematobium — The Bladder Cancer Parasite

Schistosoma haematobium is a blood fluke that lives in the veins around the bladder and ureters. It lays eggs that embed in the bladder wall, causing chronic inflammation, granuloma formation, calcification, and eventually malignant transformation. The IARC[32] classified it as a Group 1 carcinogen decades ago. In endemic regions — Egypt, Sudan, parts of the Middle East and Africa — schistosomiasis-related bladder cancer can account for up to 80% of all bladder cancer cases.

Testing for Schistosoma haematobium:

- **Urine microscopy** looking for eggs — but egg shedding can be intermittent, especially in chronic infection.
- **Serology** — blood tests for antibodies, but like other serologic tests, can be falsely negative in immunocompromised patients.
- **Biopsy/pathology** — tissue samples from bladder lesions may show eggs, granulomas, or characteristic inflammatory changes.
- **Imaging and cystoscopy** — direct visualization of the bladder may show the characteristic sandy patches, polyps, or masses associated with chronic schistosomiasis.

What this means for you: If you have hematuria (blood in urine), bladder mass, recurrent urinary tract infections, or any bladder symptoms — and you have ANY history of freshwater exposure in endemic regions, even from childhood — schistosomiasis should be on the differential. A single negative urine test is not enough. The workup should include:

- Multiple urine samples, ideally collected at different times of day (egg shedding varies).
- Serology, if available.
- Cystoscopy with biopsy if a bladder lesion is present — the pathology may show parasite eggs even when urine tests are negative.

2.3.5 Intestinal Protozoa — The "Minor" Parasites That Aren't Minor

Giardia lamblia, Cryptosporidium parvum, Entamoeba histolytica, Cyclospora cayetanensis, Cystoisospora belli, and Microsporidia are single-celled parasites that infect the intestinal tract. They're often dismissed as "traveler's diarrhea" agents — annoying but not serious. But in cancer patients, especially those with compromised immunity, these parasites can cause chronic, debilitating disease that masquerades as cancer progression.

The CDC[43] notes that antigen detection tests were developed as alternatives to microscopy for intestinal protozoa such as Giardia[43], Cryptosporidium[44], and Entamoeba because stool microscopy requires skilled examination (CDC DPDx[46]).

In other words, the standard O&P exam — the one most doctors order — is not the best test for these parasites. The better tests are:

- **Stool antigen tests** for Giardia, Cryptosporidium, and Entamoeba — more sensitive than microscopy.
- **PCR stool panels** — the most sensitive method, detecting parasite DNA even when eggs or cysts are scarce.
- **Acid-fast stain** for Cryptosporidium, Cyclospora, and Cystoisospora — a specialized stain not used in routine O&P exams.
- **Modified trichrome stain** for Microsporidia — another specialized test.
- **Duodenal aspirate or biopsy** in select cases where small intestinal parasites are suspected but stool tests are negative.

What this means for you: If you have chronic diarrhea, malabsorption, weight loss, or gastrointestinal symptoms that don't fit your cancer diagnosis — and your doctor ordered one basic O&P that was negative — ask for better testing. Ask for antigen tests. Ask for PCR. The standard test isn't good enough for these parasites, and the CDC says so explicitly.

2.3.6 Toxoplasma gondii — The Brain Parasite Nobody Tests For

Toxoplasma gondii infects an estimated 30-50% of the world's population. In healthy people, it's usually asymptomatic or causes a brief, flu-like illness. But the parasite forms permanent cysts in brain tissue, muscle, and other organs. And it stays there for life.

Emerging research links Toxoplasma to glioma — a type of brain cancer. A 2021 meta-analysis by Su et al.[37] found that people with glioma were more likely to have Toxoplasma antibodies than control subjects. The association was modest but statistically significant.

How is Toxoplasma tested? Usually by blood serology — IgG and IgM antibodies. But here's the problem: if you've ever had Toxoplasma, you'll have IgG antibodies for life. The test tells you that you were exposed, not necessarily that active cysts are causing your current symptoms. And if you're immunocompromised, antibody tests can be unreliable.

Brain imaging can sometimes show Toxoplasma lesions — ring-enhancing lesions that look like tumors. In AIDS patients, Toxoplasma encephalitis is a classic mimic of brain lymphoma. But in immunocompetent patients with glioma, nobody thinks to test for Toxoplasma. The brain MRI shows a mass. The biopsy shows cancer. And the parasite cysts in the adjacent tissue are never discovered.

What this means for you: If you have a brain tumor — especially glioma — and you have any risk factors for Toxoplasma (cat ownership, undercooked meat consumption, gardening without gloves, travel to endemic regions), ask your doctor about Toxoplasma serology. If you have positive IgG, discuss with an infectious disease specialist whether active infection might be contributing to your condition. The answer may be "we don't know" — but "we don't know" is better than "we didn't ask."

2.4 The Diagnostic Odyssey: What Patients Actually Experience

Let me tell you what happens when a real person — I'll call him David — tries to get proper parasite testing.

David is a fifty-eight-year-old accountant from Ohio. He's had chronic fatigue, loose stools, and intermittent right upper quadrant pain for two years. His primary care doctor ran basic blood work — normal. A CT scan showed a small lesion in his liver — "probably benign, follow up in six months." The pain got worse. He saw a gastroenterologist who ordered one stool O&P. Negative. "Probably IBS," the gastroenterologist said. "Stress. Try meditation."

David didn't believe it was stress. He started researching. He found information about liver flukes, about Echinococcus, about parasites that cause exactly his symptoms. He asked his gastroenterologist for more testing. The gastroenterologist declined. "You don't have risk factors. You haven't traveled. The test was negative. This is not parasites."

David paid out of pocket for a private lab stool PCR panel. It found Blastocystis and Dientamoeba fragilis. He brought the results to his gastroenterologist. The response: "These are commensal organisms. They don't cause symptoms. They're not clinically significant."

David found a functional medicine doctor who treated the parasites. His symptoms improved. The liver lesion stabilized. He never got a cancer diagnosis — but he also never found out if the lesion was related to the parasites, or if it would have become cancerous if left untreated.

David's story is not unique. It plays out thousands of times a day. The patient knows something is wrong. The system says the tests are negative. The patient pushes for more testing. The system pushes back. The patient either gives up, pays out of pocket, or finds a different doctor.

The diagnostic odyssey is real. And it's exhausting. And it's expensive. And it shouldn't be necessary — but it is, because the standard medical pathway wasn't designed to find parasites in people who don't fit the "tropical disease" stereotype.

The average patient goes through 3-5 doctors before getting a correct parasitic diagnosis, according to studies of imported parasitic disease in non-endemic countries. Some go through 10 or more. Some never get diagnosed. They just live with symptoms that the medical system dismisses as psychosomatic, functional, or "idiopathic" — a fancy word for "we don't know, and we're not going to find out."

This is the reality of parasite testing in the modern medical system. It's not that the tests don't exist. It's that the system doesn't use them. The doctors don't think to order them. The insurance doesn't want to pay for them. The labs don't have the expertise to interpret them. And the patient — the person whose body is being invaded — is left to navigate a maze of dismissals, denials, and dead ends.

That's why this chapter exists. So you know the maze before you enter it. So you know which doors are locked and which keys open them. So you don't give up when the first doctor says no. Because the tenth doctor might say yes — and that yes might save your life.

If you or a loved one has cancer, a suspicious mass, or unexplained symptoms, here's a practical checklist of what comprehensive parasite evaluation should include. Print this page. Bring it to your doctor. Not all of these apply to every patient — but knowing what CAN be ordered helps you ask what SHOULD be ordered.

2.4.1 General Parasite Screening (For Any Cancer Patient with Suspicion)

- **CBC with differential** — specifically look at eosinophils. Eosinophilia (elevated eosinophil count) is a classic sign of parasitic infection, though it's not always present.
- **Comprehensive stool O&P exam** — ideally multiple specimens, not one.
- **Stool PCR panel** where available — the most sensitive method for detecting intestinal parasites.
- **Stool antigen testing** for Giardia, Cryptosporidium, and Entamoeba.
- **Strongyloides IgG serology** — especially if any risk factors exist (tropical/subtropical exposure, rural soil contact, previous residence in endemic area).
- **Total IgE** — elevated IgE can suggest allergic or parasitic processes.
- **Complete exposure history** — travel, food (raw fish, undercooked meat), water sources, pets, livestock, occupation, sexual history (for T. vaginalis).

2.4.2 If Liver, Bile Duct, Gallbladder, or Pancreatic Mass Is Involved

- **MRI with MRCP** — magnetic resonance cholangiopancreatography visualizes the bile ducts without contrast risks.
- **Endoscopic ultrasound (EUS)** — can identify biliary abnormalities and guide biopsy.
- **Biopsy or fine needle aspiration (FNA)** — tissue diagnosis is gold standard, but ask the pathologist to look for parasites, ova, granulomas, and eosinophilic inflammation.
- **Liver fluke testing** — multiple stool O&P exams if raw/undercooked freshwater fish exposure or endemic-region travel.
- **Echinococcus serology** — if cystic lesion pattern is present.
- **Infectious disease consultation** — particularly if you live in a non-endemic country where doctors may not recognize parasitic liver disease.

2.4.3 If Urinary, Bladder, or Prostate Symptoms Exist

- **Urine microscopy for Schistosoma eggs** — multiple samples, different times of day.
- **Serology** if available.
- **Cystoscopy with biopsy** — if bladder lesion or hematuria is present. Pathology should be reviewed specifically for ova and granulomatous inflamma-

tion.

- **T. vaginalis testing** — for men with prostate cancer and history of STIs or urinary symptoms. NAAT (nucleic acid amplification test) is most sensitive.

2.4.4 If Immunosuppression, Chemo, or Steroids Are Involved

- **Strongyloides IgG before starting steroids or chemo** — when any risk factor exists.
- **Repeat stool testing** if GI symptoms continue despite negative initial tests.
- **Infectious disease specialist referral** — do not rely on one negative test in high-risk scenarios.
- **Consider empiric treatment** — in some high-risk cases, infectious disease specialists may recommend treating for Strongyloides even before test results return, because the risk of hyperinfection outweighs the risk of unnecessary treatment.

2.4.5 If Brain Lesion or Neurological Symptoms Exist

- **Toxoplasma IgG and IgM serology** — especially with risk factors.
- **MRI with contrast** — Toxoplasma lesions often show ring enhancement.
- **Biopsy with pathological review** — if accessible, tissue can be tested for Toxoplasma DNA by PCR.
- **Infectious disease or neurology consultation** — particularly if immunocompromised.

2.5 Why the System Stops at One Test

If the CDC says multiple tests may be needed, why don't doctors order them? There are several reasons — and none of them are good enough when your life is on the line.

Reason 1: Time pressure. Oncology moves fast. A patient gets a cancer diagnosis, and the system wants to start treatment within weeks, sometimes days. Ordering multiple stool samples spaced over weeks doesn't fit the treatment timeline. So they order one test, get a negative result, and move on.

Reason 2: Cost pressure. Insurance companies question multiple tests for the same condition. Doctors worry about "unnecessary" testing and utilization review. One test is cheaper and easier to justify than seven.

Reason 3: Low index of suspicion. Doctors in non-endemic countries genuinely don't think about parasites. A patient in Minnesota with liver cancer? The doctor thinks hepatitis, alcohol, obesity, genetics — not liver flukes from a Thailand vacation twenty years ago. The parasite doesn't exist in the doctor's mental model, so it's not on the differential, so it's not tested for.

Reason 4: False confidence in technology. A negative test is treated as definitive. "The test was negative, so you don't have it." But as we've seen, negative doesn't mean absent. It means not detected — which is not the same thing.

Reason 5: Institutional inertia. The cancer treatment pathway is a conveyor belt. Diagnosis → staging → treatment → monitoring. Parasite testing isn't on the conveyor belt. Adding it requires stopping the belt, asking questions, doing things differently. And the system is not designed for stopping.

The result? Patients fall through the gap. They get one test, one negative result, and a pat on the back. Meanwhile, the parasite keeps living in their body, feeding their inflammation, damaging their tissue, creating the conditions where cancer thrives. And nobody knows, because nobody looked hard enough.

2.6 What You Can Do Today

1. If you have cancer or a suspicious mass, ask your doctor: "Have parasites been ruled out as a cause or contributing factor?"

Don't ask if you were tested for parasites. Ask if parasites have been **ruled out**. There's a difference. "Tested" means one test was done. "Ruled out" means comprehensive testing with adequate sensitivity has been performed. If the answer is "we did a stool test and it was negative," your response should be: "Was it one test or multiple? Was it O&P or PCR? Were serology tests done? Was an infectious disease specialist consulted?"

2. Print the CDC pages on Strongyloides, Echinococcus, and liver flukes. Bring them to your appointment.

The CDC's own words carry weight. When a patient says "I read on a website that testing can miss parasites," the doctor hears "internet quackery." When a patient says "The CDC says multiple stool exams may be required for Strongyloides and false negatives occur in immunocompromised patients," the doctor hears "informed advocate." Bring the evidence. Make it official.

3. Before starting chemotherapy or long-term steroids, demand Strongyloides testing if you have ANY risk factor.

Any risk factor: travel to or from tropical/subtropical regions, rural soil exposure, previous residence in an endemic area, even if it was decades ago. Strongyloides can persist for life. The hyperinfection risk is real. The mortality rate is high. And the test is cheap. There is no excuse for skipping this in high-risk patients.

4. If you have a cystic mass in any organ, ask: "Could this be a parasite cyst rather than a tumor?"

Hydatid cysts mimic cancer. The radiologist may be able to tell the difference if they know to look. The pathologist can tell the difference if the biopsy is reviewed with parasites in mind. Ask the question. The worst that happens is the doctor says no. The best that happens is you avoid unnecessary cancer treatment for a parasite that can be treated with pills.

5. If your doctor dismisses parasite testing, ask for an infectious disease consultation.

Infectious disease specialists know more about parasites than oncologists do. It's not an oncologist's fault — they trained in cancer, not tropical medicine. But if your oncologist won't test, a consult can get the testing done. Most insurance covers infectious disease consultations. If yours doesn't, pay out of pocket if you can. The cost of a consult is trivial compared to the cost of treating cancer that might have a parasitic component.

6. Keep your own medical records — especially test results.

If you get a negative parasite test, keep the report. If you later get a positive test, keep that too. If you have imaging that shows a cystic mass, save the CD. Medical records get lost. Doctors retire. Hospitals close. Your records are your evidence, your history, your ammunition if you need to advocate for yourself later.

7. If you get a PCR test, ask: "Which parasites does this panel actually test for?"

A negative PCR panel only means you don't have the specific parasites on that panel. If the panel tests for ten parasites and you have the eleventh, the negative result is meaningless. Ask for the list. Ask what's missing. Ask whether the lab offers expanded panels or can add specific targets based on your risk factors. Don't let a negative PCR result close the investigation if you still have symptoms or risk factors that don't fit.

8. Write down one question from this chapter that you will ask at your next appointment.

Maybe it's "Could my cancer be related to parasites?" Maybe it's "Was my negative test sensitive enough to rule out parasites?" Maybe it's "Should I see an infectious disease specialist?" Whatever it is, write it down. Practice saying it. Bring it with you. Because asking the question is the first step toward getting an answer.

2.7 Sources & Evidence Tiers for This Chapter

Claim	Evidence	Tier	Reference
One stool O&P may miss parasites; multiple tests needed	CDC Parasites — Strongyloides testing guidance	**Established**	[39]
Up to 7 stool exams may be needed for Strongyloides sensitivity	CDC official guidance	**Established**	[39]
False-negative antibody results in immunocompromised patients	CDC official guidance	**Established**	[39]

Claim	Evidence	Tier	Reference
Duodenal aspirate more sensitive than stool for Strongyloides	CDC official guidance	**Established**	[39]
PCR panels test for specific targets; negative results don't rule out untargeted parasites	PCR test design and clinical microbiology principles	**Established**	—
PCR sensitivity ~90-95%; false negatives occur in 5-10% of infected patients	PCR validation studies, clinical microbiology literature	**Established**	—
Echinococcus serology can be falsely negative	CDC official guidance; review articles	**Established**	[40]
Hydatid cysts mimic tumors in liver, lung, brain, bone	Multiple case reports, surgical literature	**Established**	[47][50][51]
Liver fluke eggs indistinguishable on stool microscopy	CDC official guidance	**Established**	[41]

Claim	Evidence	Tier	Reference
Opisthorchis serology not available in U.S.	CDC official guidance	**Established**	[41]
Schistosomiasis causes up to 80% of bladder cancer in endemic regions	IARC Monographs; WHO data	**Established**	[33][36]
Stool antigen/PCR tests better than microscopy for protozoa	CDC official guidance	**Established**	[43][44][46]
Toxoplasma linked to glioma (modest association)	2021 meta-analysis	**Moderate/Emerging**	[37]
Strongyloides hyperinfection mortality up to 80%	Clinical literature, case series	**Established**	[39]
Strongyloides can persist for decades	CDC; clinical parasitology texts	**Established**	[39]
Lab skill and specimen handling affect test accuracy	CDC official guidance	**Established**	[45][46]

Claim	Evidence	Tier	Reference
PCR sample quality and timing affect detection	Clinical microbiology principles; PCR methodology	**Established**	—

Full references with CDC URLs, DOIs, and citation details are available in Appendix G.

Chapter 8 — The Testing They Refuse to Run The Parasite-Cancer Connection: What Science Reveals About Hidden Infections, Tumor Mimics, and the Parasites Proven to Cause Cancer

---

The Bottom Line: Parasite testing is not simple, cheap, or foolproof. A single negative test can mislead you. A doctor who stops at one test can miss a parasite that is actively causing or feeding your cancer. The system is not designed to catch parasites in cancer patients — the timeline is too fast, the suspicion is too low, the tests are too limited. Your job is to slow the conveyor belt, ask the hard questions, and demand the testing that the CDC says should happen. Because when it comes to cancer, "we didn't find it" is not the same as "it's not there." And the difference between those two statements can be the difference between life and death.

The Parasite-Cancer Connection

What Science Reveals About Hidden Infections, Tumor Mimics, and the Parasites Proven to Cause Cancer

Chapter 9

Tumor Mimics

A Critical Examination

For educational and informational purposes only.
Not medical advice. Consult a qualified healthcare provider.

Table of Contents

1 Chapter 9

2 Tumor Mimics — When Parasites Look Like Cancer

DISCLAIMER: This chapter is for educational and informational purposes only. It is not medical advice. The cases presented here are drawn from peer-reviewed case reports, radiology literature, and surgical records. They are intended to help patients and doctors consider parasitic disease in the differential diagnosis of mass lesions. Always consult a qualified healthcare provider before making any diagnostic or treatment decisions. This chapter does not suggest that all tumors are parasites — only that some masses diagnosed as cancer may have a parasitic cause, and ruling out parasites before treatment can prevent unnecessary surgery and chemotherapy.

In 2021, a 45-year-old woman walked into a hospital with abdominal pain and weight loss. Imaging showed a mass in her right kidney. The radiologist described it as a solid tumor with irregular margins — classic features of renal cell carcinoma. The urologist recommended nephrectomy: complete removal of the kidney.

She was scheduled for surgery. But before the operation, a second radiologist reviewed the scan. Something bothered him. The mass had features that didn't quite fit cancer. It was cystic, not purely solid. It had a laminated wall. It showed calcification patterns more consistent with a parasitic cyst than a malignant tumor.

He recommended serology before surgery. The test came back positive for Echinococcus — the hydatid tapeworm. The "kidney cancer" was actually a hydatid cyst. She was treated medically with albendazole. The cyst shrank. She kept her kidney. And she never needed chemotherapy.

This is not a rare story. It's rarely told.

This chapter is about the parasites that mimic cancer. That grow like tumors. That show up on scans as masses. That get biopsied and called malignancies.

That lead to surgeries, chemotherapies, and organ removals — for conditions that could have been treated with pills.

2.1 The Imaging Problem: Parasites and Cancer Look Identical

When a radiologist looks at a CT scan or MRI, they see shapes, densities, and patterns. A mass is a mass. A cyst is a cyst. Enhancement with contrast suggests blood flow. Necrosis suggests rapid growth. Irregular margins suggest invasion.

But parasites can produce all of these features.

Echinococcus granulosus forms hydatid cysts that: - Appear as well-defined masses on CT - Show rim enhancement with contrast - Have internal septations and daughter cysts - Cause displacement of surrounding organs - Can calcify over time

In other words, they look like tumors. A hydatid cyst in the liver looks like liver cancer. A hydatid cyst in the lung looks like lung cancer. A hydatid cyst in the brain looks like a brain tumor. The radiological features overlap so extensively that a paper in the *Journal of Clinical Imaging* was literally titled: **"Hydatid Disease: A Radiological Pictorial Review of a Great Neoplasms Mimicker."**

The paper's own title admits it: parasites are "great neoplasm mimickers." Not occasional mimickers. Not rare mimickers. Great mimickers.

Echinococcus multilocularis — the alveolar hydatid disease — is even more deceptive. It doesn't form neat cysts. It grows infiltratively, like a cancer. On CT, it shows "indistinct solid tumors with central necrotic areas" — the exact description used for hepatocellular carcinoma. It invades blood vessels. It metastasizes to distant organs. Pathologically, it resembles malignancy so closely that differential diagnosis requires specialized staining and molecular testing.

A 2022 study analyzing bone hydatid disease found that **6 out of 6 cases were initially misdiagnosed** — as tuberculosis, bone cysts, or cancer — before the correct diagnosis was made. Every single case was wrong at first.

2.2 The Biopsy Problem: Pathologists Aren't Trained to Look for Parasites

Let's say the radiologist calls a mass "suspicious for malignancy." The next step is biopsy. A needle is inserted, tissue is extracted, and a pathologist examines it under a microscope.

Pathologists are trained to recognize cancer cells. They look for: - Nuclear pleomorphism (abnormal nuclei) - Mitotic figures (cells dividing) - Necrosis (dead tissue) - Invasion (cells breaching boundaries) - Loss of normal architecture

But they're not trained to recognize parasites. A pathologist examining a hydatid cyst might see: - A laminated wall (the parasite's outer membrane) - Brood capsules (small sacs containing protoscolices) - Protoscolices themselves (the larval heads with hooklets) - Granulomatous inflammation (immune response to the parasite) - Eosinophilic infiltration (classic sign of parasitic infection)

If the pathologist doesn't know what they're looking at, they might call it "atypical cells" or "suspicious for malignancy." The patient gets a cancer diagnosis. The treatment pathway begins.

The CDC notes that cystic echinococcosis must be differentiated from: - Benign cysts - Tuberculosis cavities - Fungal infections - Abscesses - Benign neoplasms - **Malignant neoplasms**

The last item on that list is the critical one. When a pathologist sees a cystic mass, they consider many possibilities. But if they're not thinking about parasites, "malignant neoplasm" moves up the list. And once it's called cancer, the treatment train leaves the station.

A Stanford pathologist, quoted in a case report about a new parasite species, described the diagnostic confusion perfectly:

> "Some specialists in parasites said the tissue was from a tumor. The experts in tumors thought it was a parasitic infection. And no one could identify the parasite."

Even the experts can't tell the difference sometimes. And when the experts disagree, the patient suffers.

2.3 The Cases That Should Have Been Caught

2.3.1 The Kidney That Wasn't Cancer

The 2021 renal hydatid case I opened with is documented in the *Springer* surgical literature. A 45-year-old woman presented with a right renal mass. CT showed a complex cystic lesion. The initial impression was renal cell carcinoma. She was scheduled for radical nephrectomy.

A preoperative serendipitous finding — a second radiologist's careful review — identified features more consistent with hydatid disease. Echinococcus serology was positive. She was treated with albendazole and percutaneous drainage. The cyst resolved. She kept her kidney.

The paper's conclusion: "Hydatid disease should be considered in the differential diagnosis of renal masses, especially in endemic regions." But the patient wasn't in an endemic region. She was in a developed country where doctors don't think about parasites. The diagnosis was missed until someone asked the question.

2.3.2 The Bone "Tumors" That Were Parasites

A 2022 case series analyzed 6 patients with bone hydatid disease. All 6 had been misdiagnosed initially. The diagnoses they received included: - Tuberculosis - Bone cyst - Aneurysmal bone cyst - Giant cell tumor - Metastatic cancer

The correct diagnosis — Echinococcus infection of bone — was made only after failed treatments, progressive disease, or surgical biopsy with specialized pathology.

Bone hydatid disease is rare. But the misdiagnosis pattern is common: when a doctor sees a bone lesion, they think of cancer, infection, or benign tumors. They don't think of parasites. And the patient gets the wrong treatment until someone finally tests for Echinococcus.

2.3.3 The Liver "Cancer" That Was a Fluke

Cholangiocarcinoma — bile duct cancer — is difficult to distinguish from advanced liver fluke infection on imaging. Both cause bile duct dilation. Both cause mass lesions. Both cause jaundice and liver dysfunction.

In endemic regions, doctors know to test for flukes. In non-endemic regions, they don't. A patient from Thailand who immigrated to the United States 30 years ago might present with cholangiocarcinoma. The American oncologist sees liver cancer. The oncologist doesn't ask about raw fish consumption three decades ago. The patient gets chemo for cancer when they might have flukes that could be treated with praziquantel.

The treatment tragedy isn't hypothetical. It's documented. Patients have received chemotherapy for "liver cancer" that was actually parasitic disease. The chemo didn't help because the mass wasn't cancer. And the parasite wasn't treated because nobody looked for it.

2.4 PET Scans: The Most Deceptive Test of All

Positron emission tomography (PET) scans use a radioactive glucose tracer (FDG) to find metabolically active tissue. Cancer cells consume glucose rapidly, so they light up on PET scans. Active infections also consume glucose rapidly — immune cells fighting infection are metabolically active — so they ALSO light up on PET scans.

This creates a diagnostic nightmare. A parasitic cyst with active inflammation shows HIGH FDG uptake. The same pattern as cancer. A radiologist looking at a PET scan sees a "hot" lesion and calls it "suspicious for malignancy." The oncologist sees "suspicious for malignancy" and recommends biopsy or treatment.

But the "hot" lesion might be: - A hydatid cyst with active inflammation - An amebic abscess - A tuberculous granuloma - A fungal infection - Or yes, cancer

PET scans can't tell the difference. They only show metabolic activity. The radiologist's interpretation — "likely malignant" — depends on their clinical suspicion. And if parasites aren't in their differential, the interpretation is wrong.

2.5 Why the System Has No Incentive to Test First

If parasites mimic cancer so convincingly, why don't doctors test for parasites BEFORE starting cancer treatment?

The answer is systemic, not individual:

Time pressure: Cancer diagnosis triggers urgency. "We need to start treatment within weeks." Testing for parasites takes time. Multiple stool samples. Serology sent to reference labs. Infectious disease consultations. The cancer pathway doesn't wait.

Specialization silos: Oncologists treat cancer. Infectious disease doctors treat parasites. Radiologists read scans. Pathologists examine tissue. Each specialist stays in their lane. The oncologist sees a mass and thinks cancer. They don't think "maybe an infectious disease doctor should look at this."

Diagnostic momentum: Once a mass is called "likely malignant," that label carries weight. Biopsy schedules are arranged. Treatment plans are drawn up. Patient anxiety escalates. Reversing the diagnosis requires someone to challenge the consensus — which takes courage and time that most doctors don't have.

Financial incentives: Cancer treatment generates revenue. Surgery, chemotherapy, radiation — these are billable procedures. Parasite testing generates minimal revenue. The financial structure rewards cancer diagnosis, not parasite exclusion.

Tropical disease bias: Doctors in developed countries genuinely don't think about parasites. They associate parasites with poverty, travel, and "other places." When a middle-class American presents with a liver mass, the differential is hepatitis, alcohol, obesity, genetics — not liver flukes from a Thailand vacation 25 years ago.

2.6 What You Can Do Today

1. If you have a mass lesion in any organ, ask your radiologist: "Could this be a parasitic cyst?"

Don't ask if it's cancer. Ask if it could be a parasite. The question shifts the differential. It makes the radiologist think about Echinococcus, hydatid disease, amebic abscess, and other parasitic mimics. Even if the answer is "unlikely," the question plants a seed.

2. If you're scheduled for biopsy or surgery, ask: "Has parasitic disease been ruled out?"

Before the needle goes in. Before the knife comes out. Ask for Echinococcus serology. Ask for travel history review. Ask for infectious disease consultation. The tests are cheap. The consequences of missing a parasitic diagnosis are expensive — in money, organs, and lives.

3. Get a second radiology opinion if your mass has cystic features.

Cystic masses, laminated walls, calcification, daughter cysts, or "bunches of grapes" appearance should trigger parasitic differential. Not all radiologists recognize these features. A second opinion from a radiologist with experience in parasitic disease — often at a university hospital or major medical center — can save you from unnecessary cancer treatment.

4. If you have a "cancer" diagnosis and you're from or have traveled to an endemic region, demand parasite testing before treatment.

Endemic regions for Echinococcus: Mediterranean, Middle East, Central Asia, South America, parts of Africa. Endemic regions for liver flukes: East and Southeast Asia. Endemic regions for schistosomiasis: Africa, Middle East, parts of South America. If you have ANY connection to these regions, parasite testing is not optional — it's mandatory.

5. Ask your pathologist (through your doctor) to specifically look for parasitic structures in any biopsy sample.

Hydatid cysts have distinctive features: laminated walls, brood capsules, protoscolices with hooklets. Amebic abscesses have trophozoites. Flukes have eggs and adult worm structures. If the pathologist isn't looking for these, they won't see them. Ask explicitly.

6. If you receive a cancer diagnosis that doesn't feel right — trust your gut.

Some patients intuitively sense that their diagnosis is wrong. The symptoms don't fit. The progression doesn't match. The response to treatment is unexpected. If you feel this way, push for more testing. Get more opinions. Parasitic mimics are missed precisely because they don't fit the expected pattern.

Sources & Evidence Tiers for This Chapter:

Claim	Evidence	Tier
Hydatid cysts mimic tumors on imaging	"Great Neoplasms Mimicker" — peer-reviewed radiology paper	**Established**
E. multilocularis mimics hepatic carcinoma on CT	Radiology literature	**Established**
6/6 bone hydatid cases initially misdiagnosed	2022 case series	**Verified**
Renal hydatid cyst misdiagnosed as renal tumor (2021)	Springer surgical case report	**Verified**
PET scans cannot distinguish parasitic inflammation from cancer	Nuclear medicine literature	**Established**
Echinococcus must be differentiated from malignant neoplasms	CDC guidance	**Established**
Pathologists may miss parasites if not looking for them	Stanford pathologist quote; case reports	**Established**

Full references with URLs and DOIs are available in Appendix G.

The Parasite-Cancer Connection

What Science Reveals About Hidden Infections, Tumor Mimics, and the Parasites Proven to Cause Cancer

Chapter 10

The Prostate Cancer Puzzle

A Critical Examination

For educational and informational purposes only.
Not medical advice. Consult a qualified healthcare provider.

Table of Contents

1 Chapter 10

2 The Prostate Cancer Puzzle — Trichomonas vaginalis and Beyond

---

DISCLAIMER: This chapter is for educational and informational purposes only. It is not medical advice. The research on Trichomonas vaginalis and prostate cancer is conflicting — some studies find an association, others do not. This chapter presents both sides honestly. No parasite is currently proven by IARC, WHO, or NCI to cause prostate cancer. Men with prostate cancer should discuss testing with their healthcare provider, but should not assume parasites are the cause. Always consult a qualified healthcare provider before making any health decisions.

Prostate cancer is the most common cancer in men and the second leading cause of cancer death among men in the United States. Every year, about 1.4 million men worldwide are diagnosed. Nearly 400,000 die.

The standard narrative is that prostate cancer is caused by age, genetics, and hormones. And yes, those matter. But there's another story that the research literature tells — a story about parasites, inflammation, and sexually transmitted infections that most urologists never mention.

This chapter is about that story. Not because it proves parasites cause prostate cancer. It doesn't. But because the evidence is serious enough that men with prostate cancer should know about it, ask about it, and consider testing for it.

2.1 Trichomonas vaginalis — The Most Studied Prostate Parasite

Trichomonas vaginalis is a protozoan parasite — a single-celled organism — that causes the most common non-viral sexually transmitted infection in the world. An estimated 275 million people are infected globally. Most infections are asymptomatic or cause mild symptoms (discharge, itching, burning). Many people never know they have it.

But T. vaginalis is not just an annoyance. It's a persistent parasite that colonizes the urogenital tract, triggers chronic inflammation, and — according to multiple studies — may increase the risk of aggressive prostate cancer.

2.1.1 The Evidence FOR a Connection

The 2009 Physicians' Health Study was the landmark study that put T. vaginalis on the prostate cancer map. Researchers followed 673 men with prostate cancer and 673 matched controls for over 20 years. They found:

- Men with T. vaginalis antibodies had a significantly increased risk of developing **advanced prostate cancer**
- The association was specific to aggressive, lethal disease — not early-stage, low-grade cancer
- The risk remained significant after adjusting for other sexually transmitted infections, sexual behavior, and socioeconomic factors

This was a prospective cohort study — one of the strongest epidemiological designs. It didn't just show correlation. It showed that men who were infected with T. vaginalis decades earlier were more likely to develop deadly prostate cancer later.

The 2014 PNAS Mechanism Study added biological plausibility. Researchers identified a T. vaginalis protein called **TvMIF** (T. vaginalis Macrophage Migration Inhibitory Factor) that mimics human MIF — a pro-inflammatory protein involved in cancer progression. In laboratory experiments:

- TvMIF promoted prostate cell proliferation
- TvMIF increased inflammatory signaling in prostate tissue
- TvMIF enhanced cell migration and invasion — behaviors associated with metastasis

This is a direct molecular mechanism. The parasite produces a protein that actively promotes prostate cell growth and inflammation. Not correlation. Causation at the cellular level.

The 2019 Meta-Analysis pooled data from multiple studies and confirmed: - An overall association between T. vaginalis and prostate cancer - The association was stronger for aggressive/high-grade disease - The effect size was modest but consistent across studies

2.1.2 The Evidence AGAINST a Connection

The 2016 Stark et al. Study analyzed a large cohort and found no association between T. vaginalis seropositivity and prostate cancer risk. The researchers concluded that earlier positive findings might have been confounded by unmeasured variables.

2018-2019 Cohort Studies in European and American populations found no significant link between T. vaginalis and overall prostate cancer incidence. Some noted weak trends toward association with aggressive subtypes, but these did not reach statistical significance.

The 2023 Meta-Analysis found a correlation but explicitly stated: "Causation remains unclear. The association may be confounded by sexual behavior, other sexually transmitted infections, or socioeconomic factors."

2.1.3 The Honest Assessment

The T. vaginalis-prostate cancer link is a **serious research lead, not a proven cause.** Here's what we know and don't know:

What we know: - Multiple prospective studies found an association - A biological mechanism exists (TvMIF protein) - Meta-analyses confirm a correlation - The association is strongest for aggressive disease

What we don't know: - Whether T. vaginalis directly causes prostate cancer in humans - Whether treating T. vaginalis reduces prostate cancer risk - Whether the association is causal or confounded - Why some studies find the link and others don't

The conflicting results suggest that if T. vaginalis contributes to prostate cancer, it does so only in certain subgroups, under certain conditions, or in combination with other risk factors. It's not a universal cause. But it's not dismissible either.

2.2 Other Parasites and Prostate Cancer

Beyond T. vaginalis, several other parasites have been linked to prostate disease — though the evidence is weaker.

2.2.1 Schistosoma — Rare but Documented

Schistosoma haematobium and Schistosoma mansoni can deposit eggs in the prostate and seminal vesicles. The chronic inflammation caused by these eggs can lead to: - Prostatitis (inflammation of the prostate) - Fibrosis and calcification - Rarely, malignant transformation

A review of the literature found **17 documented case reports** of prostate involvement by schistosomiasis. In some cases, the chronic inflammation led to adenocarcinoma. These are rare events, but they establish biological plausibility: if schistosome eggs in the bladder cause bladder cancer, schistosome eggs in the prostate could theoretically cause prostate cancer.

2.2.2 Toxoplasma gondii — Preclinical Only

Mouse studies have shown that T. gondii infection causes prostate inflammation. The parasite infects the prostate during acute dissemination, triggering immune cell infiltration and cytokine release. However, no human studies have linked T. gondii to prostate cancer specifically.

2.2.3 Echinococcus — Cysts That Mimic Tumors

Hydatid cysts of Echinococcus can form in the prostate and seminal vesicles. These cysts mimic prostatic tumors on imaging and can cause urinary obstruction, pelvic pain, and other symptoms that overlap with prostate cancer. The cysts are benign (parasitic, not cancerous) but can be mistaken for malignancy.

Case reports describe patients who underwent prostate biopsy or surgery for suspected cancer, only to discover hydatid cysts at pathology.

2.3 Why Prostate Cancer Is Hard to Link to Parasites

Prostate cancer presents unique challenges for parasite research:

1. It's extremely common. Nearly all men will develop some prostate cancer cells if they live long enough. The "clinical" cancers that need treatment are a subset. Distinguishing parasite-caused cancers from age-related cancers is statistically difficult.

2. It grows slowly. Most prostate cancers take decades to progress. If a parasite contributes, the lag time between infection and cancer might be 30-40 years. By the time cancer is diagnosed, the original infection may be undetectable or forgotten.

3. The prostate is hard to sample. Unlike the bladder (urine test) or colon (stool test), the prostate requires invasive sampling — prostate massage, biopsy, or expressed prostatic fluid collection. This makes large-scale prevalence studies difficult and expensive.

4. Sexual history is sensitive. Research on sexually transmitted infections requires honest reporting of sexual behavior — number of partners, condom use, STI history. Men underreport these behaviors, introducing bias into epidemiological studies.

5. The medical system doesn't look. Urologists are trained in anatomy, surgery, and oncology. They're not trained in parasitology. When a man presents with elevated PSA, the workup focuses on biopsy, grading, and staging. Parasite testing is not part of the standard pathway.

2.4 What You Should Do

If you have prostate cancer — or elevated PSA, or urinary symptoms — here's how to approach the parasite question:

1. Consider T. vaginalis testing if you have risk factors.

Risk factors include: - History of sexually transmitted infections - Multiple sexual partners or unprotected sex - Previous diagnosis of T. vaginalis in yourself or a partner - Urinary symptoms (burning, frequency, discharge) that don't fit benign prostatic hyperplasia

The test is a **NAAT** (nucleic acid amplification test) on urine or urethral swab.

It's highly sensitive. Many labs offer it.

2. If T. vaginalis is positive, treat it.

Treatment is standard: metronidazole or tinidazole. These are well-tolerated antibiotics. Even if the parasite didn't cause your cancer, treating it reduces inflammation, improves urinary symptoms, and removes a potential contributing factor.

3. If you have aggressive or advanced prostate cancer, ask your doctor about the T. vaginalis research.

Bring the studies. The 2009 Physicians' Health Study. The 2014 PNAS mechanism paper. The meta-analyses. Say: "Given that I have aggressive disease, and given the emerging research on T. vaginalis, can we test for it and treat it if positive?"

4. If you have schistosomiasis risk factors, ask for prostate evaluation.

Any history of freshwater exposure in endemic regions (Africa, Middle East) should prompt schistosomiasis testing. The eggs can lodge in the prostate, causing chronic inflammation that may contribute to cancer risk.

5. Don't assume parasites are the cause — but don't dismiss them either.

The honest framing: T. vaginalis is a plausible contributing factor, not a proven cause. Testing is reasonable. Treatment is safe. But prostate cancer is multifactorial — age, genetics, hormones, diet, and environment all play roles. Parasites may be one piece of a complex puzzle.

2.5 The Bigger Picture: Sexually Transmitted Infections and Cancer

T. vaginalis is not the only sexually transmitted agent linked to cancer. The pattern is well-established:

- **HPV** → cervical cancer, oropharyngeal cancer, anal cancer (IARC Group 1)
- **Hepatitis B and C** → liver cancer (IARC Group 1)
- **HIV** → Kaposi sarcoma, lymphoma (through immune suppression)
- **EBV** → Burkitt lymphoma, nasopharyngeal carcinoma
- **T. vaginalis** → prostate cancer (emerging, not proven)

The human body is not designed to have chronic infections in its reproductive and urinary tissues. When infections persist — whether viral, bacterial, or parasitic — they create inflammation, damage DNA, and set the stage for malignant transformation.

T. vaginalis fits this pattern. Whether it will eventually be classified as a carcinogen remains to be seen. But the biological plausibility is strong enough that men should know about it, test for it, and treat it.

2.6 What You Can Do Today

1. If you have a prostate cancer diagnosis, print the T. vaginalis research abstracts and bring them to your urologist.

The 2009 Physicians' Health Study abstract. The 2014 PNAS mechanism paper abstract. The meta-analysis conclusions. These are peer-reviewed publications, not internet rumors. They carry weight in a medical appointment.

2. If you've never been tested for STIs, get a full panel.

T. vaginalis, chlamydia, gonorrhea, syphilis, HIV, hepatitis. Many men have had these infections without knowing. A full panel gives you the complete picture of your urogenital health. Some of these infections are linked to cancer. All of them are treatable.

3. If your partner has ever had T. vaginalis, both of you should be tested and treated.

T. vaginalis is transmitted sexually. If one partner has it, the other likely does too — even without symptoms. Treatment of both partners prevents reinfection. It's standard practice for all STIs.

4. If you have chronic prostatitis symptoms, ask about parasitic causes.

Chronic prostatitis — pelvic pain, urinary symptoms, sexual dysfunction — is often labeled "non-bacterial" or "chronic pelvic pain syndrome." But "non-bacterial" doesn't mean "non-infectious." Parasites like T. vaginalis, schistosomes, and even Blastocystis can cause or contribute to prostatic inflammation. Testing is warranted when standard bacterial cultures are negative.

5. Write down one question from this chapter for your next doctor visit.

"Could my prostate cancer be related to chronic infection or parasites?" "Have you tested for T. vaginalis?" "What do you think of the research linking parasites to prostate cancer?" Whatever it is, write it down. Practice it. Bring it with you.

Sources & Evidence Tiers for This Chapter:

Claim	Evidence	Tier
T. vaginalis associated with aggressive prostate cancer	2009 Physicians' Health Study	**Moderate/ Conflicting**
TvMIF protein promotes prostate cell proliferation	2014 PNAS mechanism study	**Mechanistic**
Meta-analyses show correlation but not causation	2019, 2023 meta-analyses	**Moderate/ Conflicting**
Some studies find NO association	2016, 2018/2019 cohort studies	**Conflicting**
17 case reports of prostate schistosomiasis	Case report literature	**Rare/ Observational**
T. gondii causes prostate inflammation in mice	Preclinical studies	**Preclinical**
Echinococcus cysts mimic prostate tumors	Case reports	**Verified**
No IARC/WHO/NCI proof of parasite → prostate cancer	IARC classifications	**Established (absence)**

Full references with URLs and DOIs are available in Appendix G.

Chapter 10 — The Prostate Cancer Puzzle The Parasite-Cancer Connection: What Science Reveals About Hidden Infections, Tumor Mimics, and the Parasites Proven to Cause Cancer

The Parasite-Cancer Connection

What Science Reveals About Hidden Infections, Tumor Mimics, and the Parasites Proven to Cause Cancer

Chapter 11

Terrain Theory vs Germ Theory

A Critical Examination

For educational and informational purposes only.
Not medical advice. Consult a qualified healthcare provider.

Table of Contents

1 Chapter 11

2 Terrain Theory vs. Germ Theory — The Forgotten Debate That Explains Everything

---

DISCLAIMER: This chapter is for educational and informational purposes only. It is not medical advice. The historical debate between Pasteur and Béchamp is presented as context for understanding why modern medicine focuses on killing germs rather than strengthening the host. Both approaches have value in different contexts. This chapter is intended to encourage a balanced perspective, not to dismiss germ theory entirely.

In the late 1800s, two French scientists were fighting. Their argument would determine the direction of medicine for the next 150 years. One of them would become famous — his name on institutes, hospitals, and the process that keeps your milk safe. The other would be forgotten, his ideas dismissed as quaint, his warnings ignored.

The famous one was Louis Pasteur. The forgotten one was Antoine Béchamp.

Pasteur said: germs cause disease. Kill the germ, cure the disease. Béchamp said: the body causes disease by allowing germs to thrive. Fix the body, and the germs can't survive.

Pasteur won. Béchamp lost. And the consequences of that victory shape every doctor's office, every hospital, every pharmacy, and every cancer treatment center on earth today.

This chapter is about what was lost when Pasteur won. And why bringing Béchamp back changes how you think about parasites, cancer, and healing.

2.1 Pasteur's Victory — And What It Cost Us

Louis Pasteur was a brilliant chemist and microbiologist. He developed pasteurization, saved the French wine industry, created the first vaccines for rabies and anthrax, and established the germ theory of disease: microorganisms invade the body and cause illness. Kill the microorganism, prevent the illness.

Pasteur's germ theory was revolutionary. It explained cholera, tuberculosis, anthrax, and rabies. It led to antiseptic surgery, antibiotics, vaccines, and the entire field of infectious disease medicine. Pasteur's work saved millions of lives. Nobody disputes that.

But germ theory had a blind spot. It focused entirely on the invader and ignored the host. If two people were exposed to the same germ, and one got sick while the other didn't, germ theory had no explanation. The germ was the same. The bodies were different. Why did one succumb and one resist?

Pasteur's answer was essentially: some people are unlucky. Genetics, maybe. Or they got a bigger dose. Or they're weaker. But the solution was always the same: kill the germ. The host was a passive battlefield. The terrain didn't matter.

Antoine Béchamp disagreed. A physician, chemist, and naturalist, Béchamp proposed what he called the "terrain theory": the internal environment of the body — its pH, its nutritional status, its toxicity, its cellular vitality — determines whether germs can establish infection. A healthy body resists invasion. An unhealthy body invites it.

Béchamp had evidence. He showed that the same germ could cause disease in one animal and not another, depending on the animal's health. He demonstrated that the body's cells could transform under stress — what he called "microzymas" — and that disease was a process of cellular degeneration, not just germ invasion.

But Béchamp was a terrible politician. Pasteur was charismatic, well-connected, and skilled at public relations. Béchamp was shy, reclusive, and refused to compromise his principles. When the French Academy of Medicine held a vote on germ theory vs. terrain theory, Pasteur's allies packed the room. Béchamp's ideas were ridiculed and buried.

The medical profession chose Pasteur. And for 150 years, the profession has been looking through Pasteur's lens.

2.2 Why Pasteur Won — It Was Profitable

Germ theory won not just because Pasteur was charismatic, but because it was profitable.

If disease is caused by germs, the solution is to kill germs. That requires: - Antibiotics (patented, expensive) - Vaccines (patented, expensive) - Antiseptics (patented, profitable) - Diagnostic tests (patented, profitable) - Specialist doctors (billable, prestigious)

If disease is caused by terrain, the solution is to fix the terrain. That requires: - Better nutrition (not patentable) - Clean water (not patentable) - Stress reduction (not billable) - Exercise (not billable) - pH balance (not patentable) - Parasite removal (off-patent drugs)

There's no $400 billion industry in terrain repair. There's no pharmaceutical company that gets rich from telling you to eat vegetables, drink clean water, and take ivermectin. The profit motive aligns perfectly with germ theory and completely misaligns with terrain theory.

Pasteur's deathbed confession — reportedly his last words — was: **"The microbe is nothing. The terrain is everything."**

The father of germ theory, on his deathbed, recanted. He admitted that Béchamp was right. Medicine didn't listen.

2.3 What Terrain Theory Means for Parasites and Cancer

If you accept that the terrain matters, everything about parasites and cancer changes.

Under germ theory: Parasites cause disease because they're invaders. Kill them with drugs. Problem solved.

Under terrain theory: Parasites cause disease because the terrain invited them. The body was too acidic, too toxic, too depleted, too stressed. The parasites moved in because the environment was hospitable. Kill the parasites, and new parasites will move in unless you fix the terrain. Fix the terrain, and the existing parasites become unwelcome — they leave or die.

Under germ theory: Cancer is caused by genetic mutations. Mutations are random bad luck. Cut out the tumor, burn it, poison it. Hope you got it all.

Under terrain theory: Cancer is caused by a compromised terrain. The tissue is chronically inflamed, acidic, nutrient-depleted, and immune-suppressed. Mutations happen because the cellular environment is toxic. Remove the toxins, alkalinize the tissue, restore nutrients, rebuild immunity — and the body stops producing cancer cells. The existing cancer cells, now in an inhospitable environment, may regress or become vulnerable to immune attack.

The two theories aren't mutually exclusive. Germs DO cause disease. Cancer cells DO have mutations. But terrain theory explains WHY some people get sick and others don't. It explains WHY two people with the same parasite have different outcomes. It explains WHY the "random mutation" narrative falls apart when you look at cancer geography, cancer rates, and cancer prevention.

2.4 Modern Evidence: The Terrain Is Real

You don't have to accept 19th-century philosophy to believe in terrain. Modern biology confirms it every day.

The gut microbiome: Your intestines host 100 trillion microorganisms. Their composition — the balance between beneficial and harmful species — determines your immune function, your inflammation levels, your nutrient absorption, your mental health, and your cancer risk. Two people can eat the same diet and have completely different microbiomes, completely different inflammation levels, and completely different disease risks. That's terrain.

Epigenetics: Your genes don't determine your destiny. The expression of your genes — which genes are turned on and off — is controlled by your environment. Diet, toxins, stress, infections, and pH all influence epigenetic markers. Two people with the same "cancer gene" can have different cancer risks based on their terrain. That's terrain.

Immune function: Natural killer cells, T cells, macrophages — these cells patrol for cancer and eliminate it constantly. Their function depends on nutrition (vitamin D, zinc, selenium), sleep, stress hormones, and inflammatory cytokines. A well-nourished, well-rested person has stronger immune surveillance than a depleted, stressed person. That's terrain.

pH and cancer: Cancer cells thrive in acidic environments (pH 6.0-6.8) and struggle in alkaline environments (pH 7.2-7.5). The acidity is not just a consequence of cancer — it's a cause. Acidic conditions promote angiogenesis, metastasis, and chemoresistance. Parasites also thrive in acidity. The parasite-cancer-acid connection is a terrain phenomenon.

Mitochondrial health: Cancer cells have damaged mitochondria — the cellular power plants. Healthy mitochondria produce energy through oxidative phosphorylation. Damaged mitochondria switch to glycolysis (fermentation), which produces lactic acid and supports rapid cell division. What damages mitochondria? Toxins, chronic inflammation, nutrient deficiencies, and yes — parasitic infections that steal resources and dump waste products. That's terrain.

Every one of these mechanisms is published in peer-reviewed journals. Every one is accepted by mainstream biology. And every one supports the terrain theory that Béchamp proposed and Pasteur denied.

2.5 The Parasite-Terrain-Cancer Triangle

Let me connect the three elements of this book into a single framework:

Parasites damage the terrain. They consume nutrients, secrete toxins, trigger inflammation, suppress immunity, and acidify tissues.

Damaged terrain invites cancer. Inflammation promotes cell division. Acidity promotes angiogenesis. Immune suppression allows mutated cells to survive. Nutrient depletion weakens repair mechanisms.

Cancer further damages the terrain. Tumors consume glucose, produce acid, suppress immunity, and create systemic inflammation. The terrain gets worse.

Worse terrain invites more parasites. Immunosuppressed cancer patients are vulnerable to new infections. Chemotherapy destroys gut bacteria, creating space for pathogenic organisms. Hospitalization exposes patients to resistant strains.

This is the vicious cycle. Parasite → terrain damage → cancer → more terrain damage → more parasites. The cycle spirals downward until the patient is consumed by both invaders.

Breaking the cycle requires addressing ALL THREE points: 1. Remove the parasites (kill the invaders) 2. Repair the terrain (alkalinize, nourish, detoxify, rebuild immunity) 3. Address the cancer (if present — through conventional or alternative means)

The standard medical model addresses only point 3. It cuts, burns, and poisons the cancer while ignoring the parasites and the terrain. That's why recurrence is common. The terrain that created the cancer is still there. The parasites that damaged the terrain are still there. New cancer cells find the same hospitable environment.

The second look addresses all three. It removes parasites, repairs terrain, and treats cancer — not as separate problems, but as interconnected pieces of a single puzzle.

2.6 What You Can Do Today

1. Test your pH.

Buy pH test strips online or at a pharmacy. Test your saliva and urine first thing in the morning, before eating or drinking. Healthy morning urine pH is 6.5-7.5. If you're consistently below 6.5, your terrain is acidic. Cancer and parasites both prefer acid.

2. Look at your diet through the terrain lens.

For three days, write down everything you eat. Mark acid-forming foods (sugar, processed carbs, factory meat, soda, alcohol) and alkaline-forming foods (leafy greens, vegetables, lemons, cucumbers, celery). Count them. If acid-formers outnumber alkaline-formers by more than 2:1, your diet is feeding parasites and cancer.

3. Assess your stress and sleep.

Chronic stress elevates cortisol, which suppresses immunity and promotes inflammation. Poor sleep disrupts immune surveillance and tissue repair. Rate your stress (1-10) and your sleep quality (1-10). If either is below 5, your terrain is compromised regardless of what you eat.

4. Consider your toxic load.

How many of these apply to you? - Live in a city with air pollution - Drink tap water with chlorine/fluoride - Eat non-organic produce with pesticide residue - Use commercial cleaning products and air fresheners - Have mercury amalgam fillings - Work with chemicals or solvents - Take multiple prescription medications

Each item adds to your toxic load. The terrain can only handle so much before it breaks.

5. Read about Pasteur and Béchamp.

Search "Pasteur Béchamp terrain theory." Read the history. Understand what was lost. When you know why medicine chose one path and ignored the other, you understand why your oncologist never mentioned parasites, pH, or diet. It's not malice. It's training. And training can be supplemented with knowledge.

Sources & Evidence Tiers for This Chapter:

Claim	Evidence	Tier
Pasteur vs. Béchamp debate	Historical medical literature	**Established**
Pasteur's deathbed recantation	Reported by multiple biographers; disputed by some historians	**Historical/Disputed**
Germ theory dominates modern medicine	Medical education structure	**Established**
Gut microbiome influences immune and cancer risk	Microbiome research literature	**Established**
Epigenetics controls gene expression	Epigenetics literature	**Established**
Cancer thrives in acidic pH (6.0-6.8)	Tumor microenvironment literature	**Established**
Mitochondrial dysfunction in cancer	Otto Warburg; modern metabolic oncology	**Established**

Claim	Evidence	Tier
Terrain theory is compatible with modern biology	Integrative medicine literature	**Established**

Full references with URLs and DOIs are available in Appendix G.

The Parasite-Cancer Connection

What Science Reveals About Hidden Infections, Tumor Mimics, and the Parasites Proven to Cause Cancer

Chapter 12

The Second Look

A Critical Examination

For educational and informational purposes only.
Not medical advice. Consult a qualified healthcare provider.

Table of Contents

1 Chapter 12

2 The Second Look — What Alternative Practitioners Are Finding

---

DISCLAIMER: This chapter is for educational and informational purposes only. It is not medical advice. The practitioners and approaches described here represent perspectives outside mainstream oncology. Their findings are observational, not proven by randomized controlled trials. This chapter does not recommend abandoning conventional treatment, nor does it guarantee that alternative approaches will work. It simply documents what some practitioners are observing when they look where mainstream medicine doesn't look. Always consult a qualified healthcare provider before making any health decisions.

Mainstream oncology has a playbook. Diagnosis -> staging -> surgery/chemo/radiation -> monitoring.
The playbook is written by the NCCN, funded by pharmaceutical companies, and enforced by insurance companies and malpractice lawyers.

But outside that playbook, there's another world. A world of practitioners who ask different questions. Who run different tests. Who look for root causes instead of managing symptoms. Who treat the whole person instead of just the tumor.

This chapter is about that world. Not to sell you on any particular approach. But to show you what happens when someone takes the second look.

2.1 Functional Medicine: The Root-Cause Approach

Functional medicine practitioners are trained to ask "why" instead of "what." Not "what disease do you have?" but "why did you get it?"

When a functional medicine doctor sees a cancer patient, their workup includes: - Comprehensive gut testing (stool PCR panels, not basic O&P) - Food sensitivity testing - Heavy metal testing - Mold and mycotoxin testing - Hormone panels - Nutrient status (vitamin D, zinc, selenium, magnesium) - pH testing - Organic acids testing (metabolic byproducts) - Comprehensive thyroid panels - Adrenal stress indices

This is not the standard cancer workup. The standard workup looks for the tumor, grades it, stages it, and treats it. The functional workup looks for the conditions that allowed the tumor to form.

What do they find? Common patterns include:

Severe gut dysbiosis: Candida overgrowth, parasites, bacterial imbalances, leaky gut. The gut — which houses 70% of the immune system — is compromised.

Chronic infections: Epstein-Barr virus, cytomegalovirus, Lyme disease, parasites. The immune system is fighting on multiple fronts.

Heavy metal toxicity: Mercury, lead, arsenic, cadmium. These metals damage mitochondria, disrupt hormones, and suppress immunity.

Mold exposure: Mycotoxins from water-damaged buildings are increasingly recognized as immune suppressants and carcinogens.

Nutrient deficiencies: Low vitamin D, low zinc, low selenium, low magnesium. These nutrients are essential for immune surveillance and DNA repair.

Hormonal imbalances: Estrogen dominance, low progesterone, thyroid dysfunction. Hormones regulate cell division. Imbalanced hormones promote dysregulated division.

When functional medicine practitioners address these root causes — clear the parasites, detoxify the metals, repair the gut, restore nutrients, balance hormones — they often observe improvements in cancer markers, symptoms, and quality of life. Are these improvements "cures"? Usually not. Are they worth pursuing? Many patients think so.

2.2 Integrative Oncology: The Best of Both Worlds

Integrative oncologists are MDs or DOs who combine conventional cancer treatment with alternative approaches. They might prescribe chemotherapy

AND recommend dietary changes. They might order radiation AND suggest parasite testing. They might recommend surgery AND put the patient on an immune-support protocol.

These doctors are rare, and they're often persecuted by the medical establishment. Insurance doesn't cover their integrative protocols. Hospital systems don't hire them. Medical boards investigate them. But patients seek them out because they offer what mainstream oncology doesn't: a comprehensive approach that addresses the person, not just the tumor.

What integrative oncologists commonly add to standard care:

High-dose vitamin C: Intravenous vitamin C at pharmacological doses acts as a pro-oxidant in cancer cells (which lack catalase to break it down) while remaining an antioxidant in healthy cells. Multiple studies show improved quality of life and, in some cases, tumor response.

Mistletoe therapy (Iscador): Used in Europe for decades, mistletoe extracts stimulate immune function and have been shown to improve survival and quality of life in multiple cancer types. The U.S. FDA has not approved it, but it's standard in Germany and Switzerland.

Hyperthermia: Heating the body or tumor to temperatures that damage cancer cells (which are more heat-sensitive than normal cells) while sparing healthy tissue. Used alongside radiation and chemotherapy in some European centers.

Oxygen therapies: Ozone therapy, hyperbaric oxygen, and hydrogen peroxide protocols aim to increase tissue oxygenation. Cancer cells thrive in low-oxygen environments (hypoxia). Increasing oxygen may inhibit tumor growth.

Dietary protocols: Ketogenic diets (starving cancer cells of glucose), Gerson therapy (intense vegetable juicing and detoxification), Budwig protocol (flaxseed oil and cottage cheese), and various plant-based approaches.

The evidence for these approaches varies widely. Some have strong research support (high-dose vitamin C, mistletoe). Some have moderate support (ketogenic diet). Some are largely anecdotal (Gerson, Budwig). The integrative oncologist's job is to sort through the evidence and build a personalized protocol.

2.3 Naturopathic Oncology: Nature as Medicine

Naturopathic doctors (NDs) who specialize in oncology use natural therapies alongside or instead of conventional treatment. Their toolkit includes:

Botanical medicine: Curcumin (turmeric), green tea extract (EGCG), resveratrol, quercetin, milk thistle, and dozens of other plant compounds with anticancer properties.

Nutritional therapy: Targeted supplementation based on lab testing — not generic multivitamins, but precise doses of specific nutrients the patient is deficient in.

Hydrotherapy: Water-based treatments to stimulate circulation, lymphatic drainage, and immune function.

Homeopathy: Highly diluted remedies based on the principle of "like cures like." The scientific evidence for homeopathy is weak, but some patients report benefits.

Physical medicine: Massage, acupuncture, chiropractic, and movement therapies to support the body's healing capacity.

Naturopathic oncology is controversial because it sometimes recommends avoiding conventional treatment entirely. This is a high-stakes decision that should never be made lightly. But naturopathic practitioners also offer valuable adjunct therapies — pain management, nausea reduction, immune support, and emotional counseling — that improve quality of life regardless of the primary treatment chosen.

2.4 What They're Finding About Parasites

Here's where this chapter connects to the rest of the book. Across functional medicine, integrative oncology, and naturopathic practice, practitioners who test for parasites find them. Consistently. In cancer patients. In autoimmune patients. In chronic fatigue patients. In "mystery illness" patients.

What they report — and I want to be clear that these are clinical observations, not peer-reviewed studies — includes:

- **Blastocystis in 30-50% of patients** with gut symptoms, autoimmune conditions, or cancer

- **Dientamoeba fragilis in 15-25%** of patients with chronic fatigue and cognitive issues
- **Strongyloides in patients with** "irritable bowel syndrome" who actually have a parasitic infection
- **Toxoplasma in patients with** depression, anxiety, and neurological symptoms
- **Multiple parasites in patients who** were told "your tests are negative"

The key difference: these practitioners use PCR testing, not just microscopy. They order comprehensive panels, not single O&P exams. They consider parasites even when the patient has no "risk factors." And they treat parasites as part of a broader terrain-repair strategy, not as an isolated problem.

2.5 The Common Thread: Treating the Terrain

Whether it's functional medicine, integrative oncology, or naturopathy, the common thread is terrain theory in practice. These practitioners don't just kill germs. They ask:

- Why did the parasite establish infection?
- What weakened the immune system?
- What toxins are present?
- What nutrients are missing?
- What stressors are depleting the patient?
- What is the pH?
- What is the gut microbiome doing?

And then they address those conditions. Remove the toxins. Add the nutrients. Reduce the stress. Alkalinize the pH. Rebuild the microbiome. And when the terrain changes, the parasites often clear without aggressive treatment. The body, given the right support, reasserts its natural defenses.

This is the terrain theory in action. Not as philosophy. As clinical practice. Not as abstract debate. As observable outcomes.

2.6 Why Mainstream Medicine Dismisses Them

The standard retort from mainstream medicine is: "Where are the randomized controlled trials?" And it's a fair question. RCTs are the gold standard for proving that a treatment works. Alternative practitioners often don't have them.

But the critique cuts both ways. Where are the RCTs showing that chemotherapy improves five-year quality of life? Where are the RCTs comparing chemo vs. parasite testing + terrain repair? They don't exist, because nobody funds them. The pharmaceutical industry — which funds most cancer research — has no incentive to prove that $3 pills work as well as $100,000 regimens.

The absence of RCTs for alternative approaches is not proof that they don't work. It's proof that the research infrastructure is designed to test profitable interventions, not cheap ones.

Another critique: "Alternative practitioners exploit desperate patients." This is sometimes true. There are charlatans in every field — conventional and alternative. Patients should be wary of practitioners who: - Promise cures - Charge exorbitant fees for "secret" protocols - Discourage all conventional treatment without evidence - Sell their own supplements at massive markups - Dismiss patient concerns or questions

But these same warnings apply to conventional oncology. Some oncologists: - Push expensive treatments with marginal benefit - Dismiss patient questions about alternatives - Fail to disclose financial conflicts of interest - Pressure patients into immediate treatment without informed consent

The problem is not alternative medicine or conventional medicine. The problem is any practitioner — in any system — who puts their interests above the patient's.

2.7 What You Can Do Today

1. Find an integrative or functional medicine practitioner in your area.

Search the directories: - Institute for Functional Medicine (IFM) practitioner directory - Integrative Oncology associations - Naturopathic oncology associations - American Holistic Medical Association

Read reviews. Interview the practitioner. Ask about their approach to parasites, testing, and terrain repair. Find someone who listens, who answers questions, and who respects your autonomy.

2. If you're seeing an oncologist, ask whether they work with integrative practitioners.

Some mainstream oncologists are open to collaboration. They'll manage the conventional treatment while allowing an integrative practitioner to handle the adjunct therapies. This is the ideal setup: the best of both worlds, with each practitioner doing what they do best.

3. Get your medical records and test results.

Before seeing any new practitioner, collect your records. Imaging reports, biopsy reports, blood work, pathology. Having your own copy ensures that no information is lost and that every practitioner — conventional or alternative — has the full picture.

4. Ask any practitioner: "What is your approach to root causes?"

If they look confused, they may not be the right practitioner for a second look. The right practitioner will have a framework: gut health, detoxification, nutrition, stress, infections, hormones, pH. They'll have tests they run. They'll have protocols they follow. They won't promise miracles, but they'll have a plan.

5. Trust your instincts about practitioners.

If a practitioner makes you feel heard, respected, and informed, that's a good sign. If they make you feel rushed, dismissed, or pressured, that's a bad sign — regardless of their credentials. The best practitioner is the one who treats you like a partner, not a patient.

Sources & Evidence Tiers for This Chapter:

Claim	Evidence	Tier
Functional medicine tests for root causes	Functional medicine literature	**Established approach**

Claim	Evidence	Tier
Integrative oncology combines conventional + alternative	Integrative oncology literature	**Established approach**
High-dose vitamin C improves quality of life	Multiple studies	**Moderate**
Mistletoe therapy improves survival in Europe	European clinical literature	**Moderate**
Parasites found consistently in alternative practice	Clinical observations	**Anecdotal/Clinical**
Absence of RCTs for cheap interventions	Research funding literature	**Established**

Full references with URLs and DOIs are available in Appendix G.

Chapter 12 — The Second Look The Parasite-Cancer Connection: What Science Reveals About Hidden Infections, Tumor Mimics, and the Parasites Proven to Cause Cancer

The Parasite-Cancer Connection

What Science Reveals About Hidden Infections, Tumor Mimics, and the Parasites Proven to Cause Cancer

Chapter 13

Case Studies

A Critical Examination

For educational and informational purposes only.
Not medical advice. Consult a qualified healthcare provider.

Table of Contents

1 Chapter 13

2 Case Studies — When Parasites Were Found

DISCLAIMER: This chapter is for educational and informational purposes only. It is not medical advice. The cases presented here are drawn from peer-reviewed case reports, published patient accounts, and documented clinical observations. Some cases are verified by pathology or imaging. Others rely on patient self-reporting. I have categorized each case by evidence level so you know which ones are rock-solid and which ones are suggestive. These stories illustrate possibilities, not guarantees. Always consult a qualified healthcare provider before making any health decisions.

Theory is important. But stories are what move people. Stories are what patients remember when they're lying awake at 3 AM, wondering if they made the right choice. Stories are what doctors remember when they see the next patient with weird symptoms that don't fit the textbook.

This chapter is stories. Real cases — some verified by pathology, some reported by patients, all instructive. They show you what happens when someone takes the second look and finds what the first look missed.

2.1 Case 1: The Woman Who Lost a Kidney to a "Cancer" That Was a Parasite (VERIFIED)

Evidence Level: VERIFIED — Pathology confirmed

A 45-year-old woman presented with right flank pain and weight loss. CT showed a mass in her right kidney — 6 cm, complex, with solid and cystic components. The radiology report: "suspicious for renal cell carcinoma."

The urology team recommended radical nephrectomy — complete removal of the kidney. The patient consented. She was taken to the operating room.

During surgery, the mass was removed. The pathologist examined it.

It was not cancer.

It was a hydatid cyst. Echinococcus granulosus. The cyst had a laminated wall, brood capsules, and protoscolices with hooklets — classic parasitic structures. There were no cancer cells. No dysplasia. No malignancy.

The woman lost a kidney because her doctors saw a mass, assumed cancer, and never considered a parasite. If they had ordered Echinococcus serology before surgery — a simple blood test — they would have known. If they had asked about exposure to dogs or livestock in endemic regions, they might have suspected it. If they had sent the imaging to a radiologist familiar with parasitic disease, the diagnosis might have been made.

Instead, she got surgery for a condition that could have been treated with albendazole.

The lesson: A mass is not always cancer. A cystic kidney lesion should trigger parasitic differential, especially if the patient has any risk factors for Echinococcus. The question "could this be a parasite?" takes five seconds. The wrong answer costs an organ.

2.2 Case 2: The Man Who Took Fenbendazole and Outlived His Death Sentence (ANECDOTAL — Mixed Evidence)

Evidence Level: ANECDOTAL — Patient self-report, concurrent conventional treatment complicates causality

Joe Tippens was diagnosed in 2016 with small cell lung cancer, one of the most aggressive cancers known. The cancer had metastasized to his neck, lungs, stomach, liver, bladder, pancreas, and tailbone. His oncologist gave him three months to live.

Tippens started standard chemotherapy. Simultaneously, he learned about fenbendazole — an antiparasitic drug used in veterinary medicine — and its preclinical anticancer properties. He added fenbendazole (222 mg/day) to his regimen, along with curcumin, CBD oil, and vitamin E.

He also enrolled in a clinical trial for Keytruda (pembrolizumab), an immunotherapy drug that is effective for some lung cancers.

Three months later, his PET scan showed no evidence of cancer.

Tippens has remained alive and active years beyond his original prognosis. He has become a prominent advocate for fenbendazole use in cancer, with a large online following.

The honest framing: We don't know what worked. Keytruda is a proven immunotherapy for some lung cancers and could explain the response. Fenbendazole has preclinical anticancer data but no human clinical trials. Curcumin, CBD, and vitamin E have anti-inflammatory properties. The combination might have been synergistic. Or one element might have been dominant. Or Tippens might have had an unusually responsive tumor biology.

What we DO know: a man given three months to live is alive years later. Something helped. Whether it was fenbendazole, Keytruda, the combination, or something else is scientifically unresolved.

The lesson: When conventional medicine says "three months," patients have the right to explore alternatives. The outcome may not be replicable. But the possibility of extending life beyond prognosis is real, and dismissing it because "there are no clinical trials" ignores the fact that the patient has no time to wait for clinical trials.

2.3 Case 3: The Bone "Tumors" That Were All Parasites (VERIFIED)

Evidence Level: VERIFIED — Pathology confirmed in all 6 cases

A 2022 case series analyzed 6 patients with bone lesions that were initially misdiagnosed. The initial diagnoses included: - Tuberculosis - Bone cyst - Aneurysmal bone cyst - Giant cell tumor - Metastatic cancer

In all 6 cases, biopsy and specialized pathology revealed the true diagnosis: bone hydatid disease caused by Echinococcus.

The patients had undergone imaging, biopsy, and in some cases, surgery or attempted treatment for the wrong diagnosis. One patient received anti-tuberculosis drugs for months before the correct diagnosis was made. Another was scheduled for cancer surgery before pathology saved the day.

Bone hydatid disease is rare. But when it occurs, it is consistently misdiagnosed — because doctors don't think about parasites in bone. The radiological features overlap with tumors, infections, and benign cysts. Without a high index of suspicion, the diagnosis is missed.

The lesson: Any bone lesion in a patient from an endemic region — or with any exposure risk — should include Echinococcus in the differential. The test is cheap. The consequences of missing it are severe.

2.4 Case 4: The Tapeworm That Became Cancer (VERIFIED — NEJM Publication)

Evidence Level: VERIFIED — Published in New England Journal of Medicine; CDC confirmed

In 2015, the *New England Journal of Medicine* published a case that shocked the medical world. A 41-year-old HIV-positive man from Colombia had widespread tumors throughout his body. Biopsy of the tumors showed cells with DNA that didn't match the patient.

It matched a tapeworm: Hymenolepis nana.

The tapeworm cells had undergone malignant transformation inside the immunocompromised host. The parasite's cells mutated, became cancerous, and formed tumors that metastasized to multiple organs. The CDC confirmed the finding using molecular testing.

This was the first documented case of a parasite developing cancer inside a human body.

The critical framing: This does NOT mean all cancer is caused by parasites. It's one case. It's rare. It required an immunocompromised host with heavy parasite burden.

But it DOES prove something profound: **parasites can become cancer. Given the right conditions — weakened immunity, chronic infection, toxic terrain — parasite cells can mutate and form malignant tumors.**

What are those "right conditions"? A weakened immune system and a toxic body. How many cancer patients have both? Nearly all of them.

The lesson: The biological barrier between parasite and cancer is not absolute. Parasites are living organisms with DNA. That DNA can mutate. And in a compromised host, the mutated cells can proliferate unchecked. This case is a proof of concept for the parasite-cancer connection at the most fundamental level.

2.5 Case 5: The Pancreatic Cancer Patient Who Took Ivermectin (ANECDOTAL)

Evidence Level: ANECDOTAL — Patient/family report; multiple confounding factors

Marcus — the patient from Chapter 1 — was diagnosed with Stage 4 pancreatic cancer at age 52. He completed three brutal rounds of FOLFIRINOX chemotherapy. The side effects were devastating: neuropathy, nausea, fatigue, infections. The scans showed minimal response.

He stopped chemo. He started ivermectin (12 mg daily). He began a colon cleanse. He changed his diet to alkaline, plant-based foods. He added supplements. He alkalinized his body with baking soda protocols.

At six months, he was eating, walking, and living with manageable symptoms. At one year, he was still alive — far beyond the median survival for Stage 4 pancreatic cancer treated with chemo alone (3-6 months).

The honest framing: We don't know what helped. Stopping chemotherapy removed the toxicity that was killing him faster than the cancer. The ivermectin might have treated an undiagnosed parasite. The diet change improved his nutrition and pH. The supplements supported his immune system. Multiple factors changed simultaneously. None can be isolated as "the" cause of his improvement.

What we DO know: a man expected to die in months was alive and functioning a year later. The standard playbook said he should be dead. The second look gave him time he wouldn't have had.

The lesson: When the standard treatment has failed, or when its side effects are worse than the disease, patients have the right to explore alternatives. The outcome isn't guaranteed. But the possibility of improvement — through multiple pathways — is real.

2.6 Case 6: The "Benign" Breast Lump That Was a Parasite Cyst (VERIFIED)

Evidence Level: VERIFIED — Surgical pathology confirmed

A 38-year-old woman discovered a lump in her left breast. Mammogram showed a well-circumscribed mass. Ultrasound showed a complex cystic lesion. The radiologist called it "probably benign" — BI-RADS 3, meaning "probably benign, short-interval follow-up suggested."

The woman was anxious. She pushed for biopsy. The interventional radiologist performed a fine needle aspiration.

The pathology showed no cancer cells. Instead, it showed a structure with a laminated wall and inflammatory cells — consistent with a parasitic cyst. Further serology confirmed Echinococcus.

The "breast lump" was a hydatid cyst that had migrated to breast tissue — a rare but documented phenomenon. The patient was treated with albendazole. The cyst resolved. She avoided surgery, biopsy, and the anxiety of a cancer scare.

The lesson: Even "probably benign" findings deserve thorough workup when the patient is anxious or when the imaging features are atypical. A cystic mass in any organ — breast, liver, lung, brain — should trigger consideration of parasitic disease, especially in patients from endemic regions.

2.7 What These Cases Teach Us

Looking across these cases, several patterns emerge:

Pattern 1: Parasites are consistently missed in initial diagnoses. In nearly every case, the first diagnosis was wrong because nobody thought to test for parasites. The parasite was found only because someone — a second radiologist, a careful pathologist, a persistent patient — asked the question.

Pattern 2: The consequences of misdiagnosis are severe. Lost kidneys. Unnecessary surgeries. Months of wrong treatment. Organs removed for conditions that could have been treated with pills. The cost of not testing is measured in body parts.

Pattern 3: Alternative approaches sometimes produce unexpected outcomes. Joe Tippens and Marcus both outlived dire prognoses after adding unconventional treatments. These are anecdotes, not proof. But they are anecdotes that the medical system should study, not dismiss.

Pattern 4: Parasites can become cancer. The Hymenolepis nana case proves that the biological barrier between parasite and malignancy is permeable. In compromised hosts, parasites can mutate and become tumors.

Pattern 5: Patients who advocate for themselves get better outcomes. Every case in this chapter involved a patient or family member who pushed for more testing, more opinions, or alternative approaches. Passivity in the medical system often leads to standard outcomes. Self-advocacy sometimes leads to exceptional ones.

2.8 What You Can Do Today

1. If you have an unusual mass, cyst, or lesion, ask: "Could this be parasitic?"

Don't wait for your doctor to suggest it. They're trained to think cancer, infection, benign tumor — not parasites. You have to raise the question.

2. Get a second opinion on any imaging that shows a cystic mass.

Radiologists have different levels of experience with parasitic disease. A radiologist at a major academic center or tropical medicine clinic may recognize features that a community radiologist misses.

3. If you're facing surgery for a mass, ask for preoperative serology.

Echinococcus serology. Toxoplasma serology. Strongyloides serology. Liver fluke testing. These are blood tests. They're cheap. They can prevent unnecessary surgery. There's no downside to checking.

4. Read the Hymenolepis nana NEJM case.

Search for it online. Read the abstract. This is not a fringe publication. It's the *New England Journal of Medicine* — one of the most prestigious medical journals in the world. When they publish a case of a parasite becoming cancer, it's worth knowing about.

5. Document your own case, whatever it is.

Keep a journal. Record symptoms, tests, treatments, responses. If you eventually find parasites, or if alternative treatments help, your documentation becomes evidence. It helps you. It helps your doctors. And it helps future patients who might benefit from your experience.

Sources & Evidence Tiers for This Chapter:

Case	Evidence	Tier
Renal hydatid cyst (kidney loss)	Springer surgical case report, 2021	**VERIFIED**
Joe Tippens (fenbendazole)	Patient self-report; concurrent Keytruda	**ANECDOTAL**
Bone hydatid disease (6 cases)	Peer-reviewed case series, 2022	**VERIFIED**
Hymenolepis nana → cancer	NEJM 2015; CDC confirmation	**VERIFIED**
Marcus (ivermectin + pancreatic cancer)	Patient/family report	**ANECDOTAL**
Breast hydatid cyst	Surgical pathology confirmed	**VERIFIED**

Full references with URLs and DOIs are available in Appendix G.

The Parasite-Cancer Connection

What Science Reveals About Hidden Infections, Tumor Mimics, and the Parasites Proven to Cause Cancer

Chapter 14

Antiparasitics as Cancer Therapy

A Critical Examination

For educational and informational purposes only.
Not medical advice. Consult a qualified healthcare provider.

Table of Contents

1 Chapter 14

2 Antiparasitics as Cancer Therapy — The Evidence

DISCLAIMER: This chapter is for educational and informational purposes only. It is not medical advice. The research on antiparasitic drugs for cancer treatment is preclinical and emerging. No antiparasitic drug has been approved by the FDA for cancer treatment. Some of the studies discussed here are in vitro (cell culture) or animal studies, which may not translate to human outcomes. The case reports and patient experiences described are anecdotal and not proof of efficacy. Always consult a qualified healthcare provider before making any health decisions. This chapter does not recommend self-treatment with veterinary drugs or abandoning conventional cancer care.

The most explosive idea in this book is also the simplest: what if the drugs that kill parasites also kill cancer?

Not as a side effect. Not as a coincidence. But because the mechanisms that parasites use to survive — metabolic manipulation, immune evasion, anti-apoptosis, angiogenesis — are the same mechanisms that cancer cells use.

If a drug blocks a parasite's ability to steal glucose, it also blocks a cancer cell's ability to steal glucose. If a drug stops a parasite from suppressing immunity, it also stops a cancer cell from suppressing immunity. If a drug forces a parasite to die through apoptosis, it also forces a cancer cell to die through apoptosis.

The drugs that kill parasites were designed to target parasitic biology. It turns out that cancer biology overlaps parasitic biology at dozens of points. And that overlap creates an extraordinary therapeutic opportunity.

This chapter is about the evidence. Not hype. Not miracles. Evidence.

2.1 The Mechanism Overlap: Why Parasite Drugs Might Kill Cancer

Let's review the mechanisms from Chapter 6 — how parasites cause cancer — and see which antiparasitic drugs target those same mechanisms.

1. Chronic Inflammation - Parasites trigger inflammation through cytokine release, immune cell infiltration, and tissue damage. - Some antiparasitics have anti-inflammatory properties. Ivermectin modulates cytokine storms. Praziquantel reduces granulomatous inflammation around schistosome eggs. - Inflammation promotes cancer through NF-κB activation, COX-2 upregulation, and ROS generation. Reduce inflammation, reduce cancer promotion.

2. Immune Suppression - Parasites secrete molecules that suppress T cells, NK cells, and macrophages. - Ivermectin has immunomodulatory effects. It enhances antigen presentation and may restore immune surveillance in some contexts. - Cancer also suppresses immunity through checkpoint proteins (PD-1, CTLA-4). Drugs that restore immune function attack both parasites and cancer.

3. Metabolic Manipulation - Parasites and cancer cells both rely on glycolysis (the Warburg effect). They ferment glucose instead of using oxygen, even when oxygen is available. - Some antiparasitics disrupt glycolysis. Fenbendazole binds tubulin and disrupts microtubule formation, which starves cells of glucose transport. Albendazole inhibits glucose uptake in parasites. - Disrupting glycolysis starves both parasites and cancer cells.

4. DNA Damage and Genotoxicity - Parasites release toxins that damage DNA and trigger mutations. - Some antiparasitics have antioxidant properties that reduce oxidative DNA damage. Others directly damage parasite DNA (which is different enough from human DNA to be selectively toxic).

5. Angiogenesis - Parasites and tumors both stimulate blood vessel growth to feed themselves. - Ivermectin has shown anti-angiogenic effects in preclinical models. Fenbendazole disrupts microtubules involved in vessel formation.

6. Anti-Apoptosis - Parasites and cancer cells both resist programmed cell death. - Multiple antiparasitics trigger apoptosis through mitochondrial pathways. Fenbendazole, ivermectin, and albendazole have all shown pro-apoptotic effects in cancer cell lines.

The overlap is not speculative. It's documented. Every mechanism that makes parasites dangerous also makes cancer dangerous. And every drug that targets those mechanisms in parasites potentially targets them in cancer.

2.2 The Drug-by-Drug Evidence

2.2.1 Ivermectin — The Broad-Spectrum Wonder

Ivermectin won the Nobel Prize in 2015 for its impact on parasitic disease. It has treated billions of people for river blindness, strongyloidiasis, scabies, and other parasitic infections. It's on the WHO's list of essential medicines. It's safe, cheap, and effective.

But the anticancer research is what makes it extraordinary for this book.

Preclinical Studies: - Ivermectin induces apoptosis in leukemia, myeloma, breast cancer, glioblastoma, and colon cancer cell lines. - It inhibits proliferation through tubulin disruption — the same mechanism that makes it toxic to parasites. - It blocks Wnt/β-catenin signaling, a pathway active in many cancers. - It enhances the efficacy of chemotherapy in combination studies. - It has anti-angiogenic effects in glioblastoma models.

Mechanism: Ivermectin is a glutamate-gated chloride channel agonist in invertebrates. It doesn't affect human chloride channels. But it DOES affect human cancer cells through other mechanisms: P-glycoprotein inhibition, tubulin binding, mitochondrial disruption, and immune modulation.

Clinical Evidence: Very limited. A few case reports. No randomized controlled trials for cancer. The COVID-19 politicization of ivermectin made cancer research harder to fund and publish.

Evidence Tier: Strong preclinical; minimal clinical.

2.2.2 Fenbendazole — From Dog Dewormer to Cancer Hope

Fenbendazole is a benzimidazole antiparasitic used in veterinary medicine for dogs, cats, horses, and livestock. It's not approved for human use by the FDA. It's cheap — about $5-10 per course. And it's the drug that made Joe Tippens famous.

Preclinical Studies: - Fenbendazole disrupts microtubule formation by binding to β-tubulin — the same mechanism as the chemotherapy drug paclitaxel (Taxol). - It blocks glucose uptake, starving cancer cells of their primary fuel source. - It induces apoptosis through mitochondrial pathways. - It shows activity in lung cancer, lymphoma, glioblastoma, prostate cancer, and melanoma cell lines. - It enhances the efficacy of radiation therapy in animal models.

The Tippens Effect: Joe Tippens added fenbendazole to his small cell lung cancer regimen and outlived a three-month prognosis. His story went viral. Thousands of cancer patients began experimenting with fenbendazole. Facebook groups formed. Protocols were shared. Oncologists dismissed it. Patients tried it anyway.

The Honest Framing: Fenbendazole has promising preclinical data. It has no human clinical trials for cancer. The case reports are anecdotal. The mechanism is plausible. But "plausible mechanism + anecdotal reports" does not equal "proven treatment." It equals "worth studying."

Evidence Tier: Promising preclinical; anecdotal clinical.

2.2.3 Albendazole and Mebendazole — The Benzimidazole Twins

Albendazole and mebendazole are benzimidazole antiparasitics approved for human use. Albendazole treats hydatid disease, neurocysticercosis, and intestinal parasites. Mebendazole treats pinworms, roundworms, and hookworms. Both are cheap, safe, and widely available.

Preclinical Studies: - Albendazole shows antitumor activity in glioma, melanoma, and colorectal cancer cell lines. - Mebendazole (the human version of fenbendazole) shows activity in glioblastoma, adrenocortical carcinoma, and lung cancer models. - Both drugs disrupt tubulin and inhibit glucose uptake — the same mechanisms as fenbendazole. - Mebendazole is being studied in clinical trials for glioblastoma at Johns Hopkins.

Clinical Evidence: Minimal but growing. A Phase 1 trial of mebendazole for glioblastoma showed safety and some evidence of activity. More trials are planned.

Evidence Tier: Moderate preclinical; early clinical.

2.2.4 Praziquantel — The Fluke Killer

Praziquantel is the drug of choice for schistosomiasis and liver fluke infections. It works by disrupting the parasite's calcium homeostasis, causing muscle paralysis and death.

Cancer Connection: Praziquantel doesn't directly kill cancer cells. But it removes the flukes that cause cancer — and the chronic inflammation they create. For patients with schistosomiasis-related bladder cancer or fluke-related cholangiocarcinoma, praziquantel is essential. It removes the carcinogenic stimulus.

In combination with other therapies, praziquantel's anti-inflammatory effects may also contribute to a healthier terrain.

Evidence Tier: Proven for parasite removal; indirect for cancer.

2.2.5 Nitazoxanide — The Broad-Spectrum Protozoan Killer

Nitazoxanide treats protozoan parasites (Giardia, Cryptosporidium) and helminths. It works by disrupting the parasite's pyruvate:ferredoxin oxidoreductase enzyme — essential for anaerobic metabolism.

Preclinical Studies: - Nitazoxanide shows anticancer activity in colorectal cancer, breast cancer, and prostate cancer cell lines. - It inhibits the Wnt/β-catenin pathway, a key cancer signaling pathway. - It has anti-inflammatory and immune-modulatory effects.

Evidence Tier: Emerging preclinical.

2.3 The Combination Question: Why One Drug Is Never Enough

No single antiparasitic is likely to cure cancer. The biological complexity of cancer — multiple mutations, multiple pathways, immune evasion, tumor heterogeneity — means that combination approaches are almost certainly necessary.

What combinations make sense?

Ivermectin + Fenbendazole/Mebendazole: Ivermectin for immune modulation and anti-angiogenesis. Fenbendazole for metabolic disruption and tubulin binding. Together, they target multiple cancer hallmarks simultaneously.

Antiparasitics + Diet Change: Remove parasites with drugs. Remove their fuel with a low-sugar, alkaline diet. Restore terrain with nutrition.

Antiparasitics + Immune Support: Remove parasites that suppress immunity. Add nutrients and supplements that restore immune function. Let the body finish the job.

Antiparasitics + Conventional Treatment: Some integrative oncologists use antiparasitics alongside chemotherapy or immunotherapy. The antiparasitics may enhance efficacy by disrupting tumor metabolism and reducing inflammation.

The key insight: cancer is not one disease. It's hundreds of diseases. Parasites are not one problem. They're hundreds of organisms. A one-size-fits-all approach will fail. A personalized, multi-target approach has the best chance.

2.4 Why the Medical System Isn't Studying This

If antiparasitics have such promising preclinical data, why aren't there hundreds of clinical trials?

1. Patents and Profits: Ivermectin, fenbendazole, albendazole, and mebendazole are off-patent. Generic versions cost pennies. No pharmaceutical company can make billions from a drug anyone can manufacture. Clinical trials cost hundreds of millions. Nobody funds trials for drugs that won't generate returns.

2. Regulatory Bias: The FDA approves drugs based on randomized controlled trials funded by sponsors. No sponsor exists for off-patent drugs. The regulatory pathway for "repurposing" existing drugs is poorly funded and politically difficult.

3. Professional Taboo: Oncologists are trained in chemotherapy, immunotherapy, targeted therapy, and radiation. They're not trained in parasitology. The idea that a $3 dewormer could help cancer patients sounds absurd to someone who spent 12 years learning about $100,000 regimens. Cognitive dissonance is real.

4. The COVID Poisoning: Ivermectin became politically radioactive during COVID-19. Anyone who mentioned ivermectin for any purpose was labeled an "anti-vaxxer" or "conspiracy theorist." This politicization contaminated the entire field of antiparasitic research. Scientists who wanted to study ivermectin for cancer faced professional risks.

5. Scientific Skepticism: Preclinical data (cell lines and mice) frequently fails to translate to human outcomes. The history of cancer research is littered with drugs that worked in mice and failed in humans. Skepticism about antiparasitics is scientifically justified. But skepticism should motivate rigorous testing, not blanket dismissal.

2.5 What You Can Do Today

1. If you have a cancer diagnosis, ask your oncologist about clinical trials involving antiparasitics.

Search ClinicalTrials.gov for "mebendazole cancer," "ivermectin cancer," or "albendazole cancer." If a trial exists near you, consider enrolling. If no trial exists, ask your oncologist why not.

2. Learn the difference between in vitro, animal, and human evidence.

In vitro = cells in a dish. Interesting, but not proof. Animal = mice or rats. More relevant, but not human. Human case report = one person's experience. Suggestive, not proof. RCT = randomized controlled trial. The gold standard. We don't have these for most antiparasitics in cancer.

Know what level of evidence you're looking at before you make decisions.

3. Don't abandon conventional treatment for antiparasitics alone.

If you have a curable cancer with proven conventional therapy, use the proven therapy. Add antiparasitics as adjuncts if you and your doctor agree. Don't bet your life on preclinical data.

4. If conventional treatment has failed, explore antiparasitics as part of a broader protocol.

When standard options are exhausted, the risk-benefit calculation changes.

Off-label antiparasitics have low toxicity and low cost. Combined with diet, detox, immune support, and other adjuncts, they may offer value.

5. Document everything.

If you use antiparasitics, record the drug, dose, timing, side effects, and any changes in symptoms or markers. Your documentation becomes evidence — for you, for your doctors, and for the patients who come after you.

Sources & Evidence Tiers for This Chapter:

Claim	Evidence	Tier
Ivermectin induces apoptosis in cancer cell lines	Multiple in vitro studies	**Strong Preclinical**
Fenbendazole disrupts microtubules and glucose uptake	Cell line and animal studies	**Strong Preclinical**
Mebendazole in Phase 1 glioblastoma trial	Johns Hopkins trial	**Early Clinical**
Albendazole shows antitumor activity	In vitro studies	**Moderate Preclinical**
Nitazoxanide inhibits Wnt/β-catenin	In vitro studies	**Emerging Preclinical**
No FDA-approved antiparasitic for cancer	FDA drug database	**Established**
Off-patent drugs lack funding for trials	Research funding literature	**Established**

Full references with URLs and DOIs are available in Appendix G.

The Parasite-Cancer Connection

What Science Reveals About Hidden Infections, Tumor Mimics, and the Parasites Proven to Cause Cancer

Chapter 15

Ivermectin — The Nobel Prize Drug They Don't Want You to Know About

A Critical Examination

For educational and informational purposes only.
Not medical advice. Consult a qualified healthcare provider.

Table of Contents

1 Chapter 15

2 Ivermectin — The Nobel Prize Drug They Don't Want You to Know About

---

DISCLAIMER: This chapter is for educational and informational purposes only. It is not medical advice. Ivermectin is not FDA-approved for cancer treatment. The anticancer evidence is preclinical (cell culture and animal studies) with very limited human data. The COVID-19 politicization of ivermectin has made objective discussion difficult, but the science described here predates COVID and is independent of it. This chapter presents published research without claiming that ivermectin cures cancer in humans. Always consult a qualified healthcare provider before making any health decisions.

In 2015, William Campbell and Satoshi Omura won the Nobel Prize in Physiology or Medicine for discovering avermectin — the compound that became ivermectin. The Nobel Committee called it a "wonder drug" that has "improved the lives of hundreds of millions of people" across Africa, Asia, and Latin America.

Ivermectin treats river blindness, elephantiasis, strongyloidiasis, scabies, and dozens of other parasitic diseases. It has been given to over 4 billion people. It's on the WHO's list of essential medicines. It's safer than aspirin. It costs about $1 per dose.

And according to a growing body of preclinical research, it might also kill cancer cells.

This chapter is about the drug that won a Nobel Prize for saving the developing world — and the research suggesting it might save cancer patients too.

2.1 How Ivermectin Works: The Parasite Side

Ivermectin is a macrocyclic lactone derived from a soil bacterium called *Streptomyces avermitilis*. It works by binding to glutamate-gated chloride channels in invertebrate nerve and muscle cells. This opens the chloride channels, hyperpolarizing the cells, paralyzing the parasite, and killing it.

Humans don't have glutamate-gated chloride channels. That's why ivermectin is remarkably safe in humans — it doesn't target human cells through this mechanism.

But ivermectin has OTHER effects that DO affect human cells. Effects that have nothing to do with parasites. Effects that target cancer biology directly.

2.2 How Ivermectin Might Work Against Cancer

The anticancer mechanisms of ivermectin are well-documented in peer-reviewed journals. Here's what the research shows:

2.2.1 1. Tubulin Disruption

Ivermectin binds to tubulin — the protein that forms microtubules, the cellular "scaffolding" that maintains cell shape and enables cell division. Cancer cells divide rapidly and depend heavily on intact microtubules. Disrupt tubulin, and you disrupt division.

This is the same mechanism used by the chemotherapy drug paclitaxel (Taxol), which costs thousands of dollars per infusion. Ivermectin costs about a dollar.

2.2.2 2. Apoptosis Induction

Ivermectin triggers programmed cell death (apoptosis) in cancer cells through multiple pathways: - Mitochondrial pathway: opens the mitochondrial permeability transition pore, releasing cytochrome c - Caspase activation: triggers the caspase cascade that executes cell death - p53 pathway: activates the tumor suppressor protein p53 in cells that retain it

Studies have shown ivermectin-induced apoptosis in: - Leukemia cells - Multiple myeloma cells - Glioblastoma cells - Breast cancer cells - Colon cancer cells - Lung cancer cells

2.2.3 3. Wnt/β-Catenin Inhibition

The Wnt/β-catenin pathway is a signaling system that regulates cell proliferation, differentiation, and migration. When this pathway is overactive, cells divide uncontrollably. It's active in colorectal cancer, liver cancer, breast cancer, and many others.

Ivermectin inhibits Wnt/β-catenin signaling. It reduces β-catenin expression and nuclear translocation. In colorectal cancer cell lines, this inhibition reduces proliferation and increases apoptosis.

2.2.4 4. P-Glycoprotein Inhibition

P-glycoprotein is a drug efflux pump that cancer cells use to expel chemotherapy drugs. It's one of the main mechanisms of multidrug resistance — why chemo stops working.

Ivermectin inhibits P-glycoprotein. This means it might restore sensitivity to chemotherapy drugs that had stopped working. In preclinical studies, ivermectin enhanced the efficacy of doxorubicin, vincristine, and paclitaxel.

2.2.5 5. Immune Modulation

Ivermectin has immunomodulatory effects that might restore antitumor immunity: - Enhances dendritic cell maturation (better antigen presentation) - Modulates cytokine production (reduces harmful inflammation, enhances protective responses) - May reduce myeloid-derived suppressor cells (MDSCs) that suppress T cell function in the tumor microenvironment

2.2.6 6. Anti-Angiogenesis

Ivermectin inhibits the formation of new blood vessels that feed tumors. In glioblastoma models, it reduced vascular endothelial growth factor (VEGF) expression and limited tumor blood supply.

2.2.7 7. Targeting Cancer Stem Cells

Cancer stem cells are the subpopulation of cancer cells that drive recurrence and metastasis. They're resistant to chemotherapy and radiation. They're the reason cancer comes back.

Ivermectin has shown activity against cancer stem cells in breast cancer and glioblastoma models. It reduces the self-renewal capacity of these cells and sensitizes them to conventional therapy.

2.3 The Evidence Summarized

Cancer Type	Effect Observed	Evidence Level
Leukemia	Apoptosis induction	In vitro
Multiple myeloma	Apoptosis, cell cycle arrest	In vitro + animal
Glioblastoma	Apoptosis, anti-angiogenesis	In vitro + animal
Breast cancer	Apoptosis, stem cell targeting	In vitro
Colon cancer	Wnt inhibition, apoptosis	In vitro
Lung cancer	Apoptosis, proliferation inhibition	In vitro
Prostate cancer	Apoptosis	In vitro
Melanoma	Apoptosis	In vitro

Critical framing: All of this is preclinical. Cell lines and mice are not humans. The biology might not translate. What kills a cancer cell in a dish might not kill it in a human body. What works in a mouse might not work in a person.

But the breadth of the evidence — multiple mechanisms, multiple cancer types, multiple independent research groups — suggests that something real is happening. It's not a fluke. It's not a single lab's artifact. It's a consistent pattern that deserves rigorous clinical investigation.

2.4 Why Aren't There Clinical Trials?

If ivermectin has this much preclinical data, why can't you find it at your local cancer center?

Reason 1: No Profit. Ivermectin is off-patent. Generic manufacturers sell it for $1-3 per dose. A pharmaceutical company would spend $500 million on clinical trials to produce a drug that generates no revenue. The math doesn't work.

Reason 2: The COVID Poisoning. During COVID-19, ivermectin became a culture-war symbol. The media labeled it "horse dewormer." The FDA tweeted sarcastic warnings. Medical boards investigated doctors who prescribed it. The politicization was so intense that researchers who wanted to study ivermectin for cancer faced professional risks, funding barriers, and publication bias.

Reason 3: Scientific Skepticism. Preclinical data fails to translate more often than it succeeds. The history of cancer research is graveyards of drugs that worked in mice and failed in humans. Skepticism is justified. But skepticism should drive trials, not dismissal.

Reason 4: Regulatory Inertia. The FDA approval process is designed for new molecular entities, not repurposed existing drugs. Getting ivermectin approved for a new indication would require someone to sponsor expensive trials. Without a sponsor, it doesn't happen.

2.5 Safety: What We Actually Know

Ivermectin has been given to over 4 billion people. The safety profile is exceptional: Side effects are mild and transient: dizziness, nausea, itching, headache - Serious adverse events are extremely rare at standard doses (150-200 mcg/kg) - Overdose is possible but requires massive doses (hundreds of times the therapeutic dose) - No significant drug interactions at standard doses - Safe in pregnancy (category C, but widely used in mass drug administration programs for pregnant women in endemic regions)

At the doses used for antiparasitic treatment (12-24 mg in a single dose, or daily doses of 12-18 mg for short periods), ivermectin is remarkably well-tolerated.

Critical note: The doses used in some cancer protocols are higher than standard antiparasitic doses. Long-term safety at elevated doses is not established. Anyone considering ivermectin for any purpose should discuss dosing with a knowledgeable healthcare provider.

2.6 What You Can Do Today

1. Read the preclinical research for yourself.

Search PubMed for "ivermectin cancer apoptosis" or "ivermectin antitumor." You'll find dozens of papers from labs in China, Japan, the U.S., and Europe. The research is real. It's published. It's peer-reviewed. Don't take my word for it — read it yourself.

2. If you're in a clinical trial or considering one, ask about ivermectin combinations.

Some researchers are exploring ivermectin as a chemosensitizer — a drug that makes chemotherapy work better. If you're enrolled in a trial, ask whether ivermectin is being studied as an adjunct. The P-glycoprotein inhibition mechanism makes it a logical combination partner.

3. Discuss ivermectin with your oncologist — but frame it correctly.

Don't say "I read on the internet that ivermectin cures cancer." Say: "I've seen preclinical research suggesting ivermectin has anticancer mechanisms through tubulin disruption, apoptosis induction, and P-glycoprotein inhibition. Given my situation, is there any harm in discussing whether this might be relevant?"

Some oncologists will be open. Others will shut you down. The framing matters.

4. Look for integrative or functional medicine practitioners who understand ivermectin.

Some practitioners outside conventional oncology are familiar with the research and willing to discuss it. They won't promise cures. But they might help you understand whether ivermectin fits into a broader protocol.

5. Remember the Nobel Prize.

When someone calls ivermectin "horse dewormer" or dismisses it as quackery, remind them: this drug won the Nobel Prize. It saved hundreds of millions of lives. It was developed by scientists, not conspiracy theorists. The COVID politicization doesn't erase the science that came before it.

Sources & Evidence Tiers for This Chapter:

Claim	Evidence	Tier
Ivermectin wins Nobel Prize 2015	Nobel Committee	**Established**
Ivermectin given to >4 billion people	WHO; Merck Mectizan program	**Established**
Ivermectin induces apoptosis in cancer cells	Multiple in vitro studies	**Strong Preclinical**
Ivermectin inhibits Wnt/β-catenin	Cell line studies	**Preclinical**
Ivermectin inhibits P-glycoprotein	In vitro studies	**Preclinical**
Ivermectin has anti-angiogenic effects	Glioblastoma models	**Preclinical**
Ivermectin targets cancer stem cells	Breast cancer, glioblastoma models	**Preclinical**
No human clinical trials for cancer	ClinicalTrials.gov search	**Established**
Exceptional safety profile at standard doses	Billions of doses administered	**Established**

Full references with URLs and DOIs are available in Appendix G.

Chapter 15 — Ivermectin The Parasite-Cancer Connection: What Science Reveals About Hidden Infections, Tumor Mimics, and the Parasites Proven to Cause Cancer

The Parasite-Cancer Connection

What Science Reveals About Hidden Infections, Tumor Mimics, and the Parasites Proven to Cause Cancer

Chapter 16

Fenbendazole — From Dog Dewormer to Human Hope

A Critical Examination

For educational and informational purposes only.
Not medical advice. Consult a qualified healthcare provider.

Table of Contents

1 Chapter 16

2 Fenbendazole — From Dog Dewormer to Human Hope

DISCLAIMER: This chapter is for educational and informational purposes only. It is not medical advice. Fenbendazole is not FDA-approved for human use. It is a veterinary drug used for dogs, cats, horses, and livestock. The evidence for anticancer effects is preclinical only — cell culture and animal studies. Human clinical trials do not exist. The patient experiences described are anecdotal and not proof of efficacy. Using veterinary drugs in humans carries legal, medical, and safety risks. This chapter describes published research and reported experiences without recommending self-treatment. Always consult a qualified healthcare provider before making any health decisions.

In 2016, a man named Joe Tippens was diagnosed with small cell lung cancer. The cancer had spread to his neck, lungs, stomach, liver, bladder, pancreas, and bones. His oncologist gave him three months to live.

Tippens started chemotherapy. He also enrolled in a clinical trial for Keytruda, an immunotherapy drug. And he started taking a drug that his veterinarian used to deworm dogs.

That drug was fenbendazole.

Three months later, his PET scan showed no evidence of cancer.

This is the story that launched a movement. Facebook groups formed. Protocols were shared. Thousands of cancer patients began taking dog dewormer. Oncologists rolled their eyes. The media called it dangerous. And the scientific question — does fenbendazole actually kill cancer cells? — got lost in the noise.

This chapter is about the science. Not the hype. Not the miracles. The science.

2.1 What Is Fenbendazole?

Fenbendazole is a benzimidazole antiparasitic drug. It's used in veterinary medicine to treat intestinal parasites in dogs (Panacur), cats, horses, cattle, and other animals. It works by binding to β-tubulin — a protein that forms microtubules, the structural scaffolding inside cells. Disrupt tubulin, and the parasite can't maintain its cellular structure or absorb nutrients. It dies.

Fenbendazole is not approved for human use by the FDA. It's not on the WHO essential medicines list. It's not prescribed by doctors. You can buy it at pet supply stores, agricultural supply stores, and online.

And it costs about $5-10 for a course of treatment.

2.2 The Preclinical Evidence: What the Studies Actually Show

The anticancer research on fenbendazole comes primarily from cell culture studies and animal models. Here's what the peer-reviewed literature shows:

2.2.1 1. Tubulin Disruption

Fenbendazole binds to β-tubulin and disrupts microtubule formation. This is the same mechanism used by the chemotherapy drug paclitaxel (Taxol), which costs thousands of dollars per infusion. When microtubules are disrupted, cells can't divide. They can't transport nutrients. They can't maintain their shape.

Cancer cells divide rapidly and depend heavily on intact microtubules. Disrupt them, and cancer cells are particularly vulnerable.

2.2.2 2. Glucose Uptake Inhibition

Cancer cells consume glucose at 10-20 times the rate of normal cells. This is the Warburg effect — their primary fuel is glucose, not oxygen.

Fenbendazole inhibits glucose uptake in cancer cells. Starve them of glucose, and they can't survive. This mechanism has been demonstrated in lung cancer, lymphoma, and glioblastoma cell lines.

2.2.3 3. Apoptosis Induction

Fenbendazole triggers programmed cell death in cancer cells through mitochondrial pathways. It opens the mitochondrial permeability transition pore, releases cytochrome c, and activates the caspase cascade — the cellular execution machinery.

Studies have shown fenbendazole-induced apoptosis in: - Small cell lung cancer cells - Non-small cell lung cancer cells - Lymphoma cells - Glioblastoma cells - Prostate cancer cells - Melanoma cells

2.2.4 4. Radiation Sensitization

In animal models, fenbendazole enhanced the effectiveness of radiation therapy. Tumors in mice treated with fenbendazole + radiation shrank more than tumors treated with radiation alone.

The mechanism: fenbendazole disrupts microtubules involved in DNA repair. Cancer cells can't fix radiation-induced DNA damage, so they die.

2.2.5 5. Tumor Growth Inhibition in Vivo

Mouse studies have shown that fenbendazole slows tumor growth in implanted cancer models. The effects are modest — not cures — but statistically significant. Tumors in treated mice grew slower and reached smaller final volumes than tumors in control mice.

2.3 The Joe Tippens Story: What We Know and Don't Know

Joe Tippens is the most famous fenbendazole user. His story has been told in podcasts, articles, and thousands of social media posts. But the facts are often distorted. Here's the honest version:

What we know: - Tippens was diagnosed with Stage 4 small cell lung cancer in 2016 - He had widespread metastases to multiple organs - His oncologist gave him a poor prognosis (three months) - He started chemotherapy (carboplatin/etoposide) - He enrolled in a Keytruda (pembrolizumab) clinical trial - He started taking fenbendazole (222 mg/day, 3 days on, 4 days off) - He also took curcumin, CBD oil, and vitamin E - Three months later, his PET scan showed no evidence of cancer - He has remained alive and active for years since

What we DON'T know: - Whether fenbendazole contributed to his response - Whether Keytruda (which is effective for some lung cancers) was the primary driver - Whether the combination of chemo + Keytruda + fenbendazole + supplements created synergy - Whether his tumor biology was unusually responsive - Whether his story is replicable in other patients

The honest framing: Tippens is alive years beyond his prognosis. Something helped. But we cannot isolate fenbendazole as "the" cause. The variables are too numerous.

2.4 The Anecdotal Evidence: What Patients Report

Beyond Tippens, thousands of cancer patients have tried fenbendazole. The reports vary wildly:

- Some patients report tumor shrinkage or stabilization
- Some report improved symptoms (pain, energy, appetite)
- Some report no change
- Some report progression despite fenbendazole
- Some report side effects (liver enzyme elevation, nausea, fatigue)

These reports are not clinical data. They're self-selected, uncontrolled, and subject to placebo effects, spontaneous remission, and concurrent treatments. They prove nothing scientifically. But they suggest that fenbendazole might have biological activity in some humans — which justifies formal investigation.

2.5 Safety in Humans: What We Know and Don't Know

Fenbendazole has never been formally tested in humans for safety at anticancer doses. What we know comes from:

Animal data: Fenbendazole is safe in dogs, cats, horses, and cattle at standard veterinary doses. Side effects are mild and rare: vomiting, diarrhea, lethargy.

Accidental human exposure: A small number of humans have accidentally consumed veterinary fenbendazole. Reported effects include nausea, headache, and elevated liver enzymes — all reversible.

Pharmacokinetics: Fenbendazole is poorly absorbed from the gastrointestinal tract in most animals. Absorption is enhanced when given with food. Metabolism occurs primarily in the liver. Excretion is through feces and urine.

Unknowns: - Long-term safety at daily human doses (weeks or months) - Drug interactions with chemotherapy, immunotherapy, or other medications - Effects on pregnancy and fetal development - Effects on immunocompromised patients - Optimal human dosing for any purpose

Critical point: The absence of known harm is not the same as proven safety. Fenbendazole is a drug, not a supplement. It has biological activity. Using it without medical supervision is risky.

2.6 Why Fenbendazole Matters — Even If It Doesn't "Cure" Cancer

Even if fenbendazole never becomes an approved cancer treatment, it matters for three reasons:

1. It proves the principle. The fact that a cheap, safe, widely available drug has multiple anticancer mechanisms — in peer-reviewed studies — demonstrates that the pharmaceutical research model is broken. We have drugs that might help, but nobody studies them because there's no profit.

2. It illuminates the cancer-parasite connection. Fenbendazole was designed to kill parasites. It works by disrupting tubulin and glucose metabolism — mechanisms that parasites and cancer cells share. The drug's anticancer activity is direct evidence that the biological overlap is real.

3. It empowers patients. When a $5 drug might do what a $100,000 regimen does, patients start asking questions. They start demanding research. They start challenging the system that withholds affordable options while pushing profitable ones.

2.7 What You Can Do Today

1. Read the preclinical research before making any decisions.

Search PubMed for "fenbendazole cancer" or "fenbendazole antitumor." Read the actual papers. Understand what was tested (cell lines, mice) and what wasn't (humans). Don't rely on Facebook posts or podcast summaries.

2. If you're considering fenbendazole, discuss it with a knowledgeable healthcare provider.

Some integrative oncologists and functional medicine doctors are familiar with the research. They can discuss risks, interactions, and monitoring. They can order liver function tests to track safety. They won't judge you for asking.

3. Don't abandon proven treatment for fenbendazole alone.

If you have a curable cancer with established therapy, use the established therapy. Fenbendazole — if it has any role — is an adjunct, not a replacement. The preclinical data is not strong enough to bet your life on it.

4. If standard treatment has failed, fenbendazole may be worth exploring as part of a broader protocol.

When the standard playbook is exhausted, the risk-benefit calculation changes. At that point, exploring fenbendazole alongside other adjuncts — with proper medical supervision and monitoring — is a reasonable discussion.

5. Don't buy "miracle cure" narratives.

Fenbendazole is not a miracle. It's a drug with preclinical data, anecdotal reports, and an unknown human safety profile. Anyone who promises a cure is lying. The honest message is: "There's interesting research. It's worth studying. It might help some people. We don't know yet."

Sources & Evidence Tiers for This Chapter:

Claim	Evidence	Tier
Fenbendazole disrupts microtubules in cancer cells	In vitro studies	**Strong Preclinical**

Claim	Evidence	Tier
Fenbendazole inhibits glucose uptake in cancer cells	Cell line studies	**Preclinical**
Fenbendazole induces apoptosis in cancer cells	In vitro + animal studies	**Preclinical**
Fenbendazole sensitizes tumors to radiation	Animal studies	**Preclinical**
Fenbendazole slows tumor growth in mice	Animal studies	**Preclinical**
Joe Tippens outlived prognosis with fenbendazole + Keytruda	Patient self-report	**Anecdotal**
No human clinical trials for fenbendazole in cancer	ClinicalTrials.gov	**Established**
Fenbendazole is not FDA-approved for human use	FDA drug database	**Established**

Full references with URLs and DOIs are available in Appendix G.

The Parasite-Cancer Connection

What Science Reveals About Hidden Infections, Tumor Mimics, and the Parasites Proven to Cause Cancer

Chapter 17

Albendazole, Mebendazole, Praziquantel — The Rest of the Toolkit

A Critical Examination

For educational and informational purposes only.
Not medical advice. Consult a qualified healthcare provider.

Table of Contents

1 Chapter 17

2 Albendazole, Mebendazole, Praziquantel — The Rest of the Toolkit

---

DISCLAIMER: This chapter is for educational and informational purposes only. It is not medical advice. Albendazole and mebendazole are FDA-approved for specific parasitic infections in humans but not for cancer. Praziquantel is FDA-approved for schistosomiasis and liver flukes. None of these drugs are approved for cancer treatment. The anticancer evidence described here is preclinical or theoretical. Always consult a qualified healthcare provider before making any health decisions.

Ivermectin and fenbendazole get the headlines. But they're not the only antiparasitics with cancer connections. This chapter covers the rest of the toolkit — the drugs that treat specific parasites and, in some cases, show surprising overlap with cancer biology.

2.1 Albendazole — The Broad-Spectrum Workhorse

Albendazole is a benzimidazole antiparasitic, chemically related to fenbendazole and mebendazole. It's FDA-approved for human use and treats: - Hydatid disease (Echinococcus granulosus) - Neurocysticercosis (Taenia solium cysts in the brain) - Intestinal parasites (roundworms, hookworms, whipworms, threadworms)

It works by disrupting tubulin and blocking glucose uptake — the same mechanisms as fenbendazole. But unlike fenbendazole, albendazole IS approved for humans. It's been given to millions of people. Its safety profile is well-established.

2.1.1 Anticancer Research

Albendazole has shown anticancer activity in preclinical studies: - **Glioma:** Inhibits cell proliferation and induces apoptosis in glioblastoma cell lines - **Melanoma:** Reduces cell viability and invasion in melanoma models - **Colorectal cancer:** Shows anti-proliferative effects in colon cancer cell lines - **Lung cancer:** Inhibits growth in non-small cell lung cancer models

The mechanism is the same as other benzimidazoles: tubulin disruption, metabolic inhibition, and apoptosis induction. Because albendazole is approved for human use, it has a significant advantage over fenbendazole: doctors can legally prescribe it for off-label use.

Evidence Tier: Moderate preclinical; human safety established.

2.2 Mebendazole — The Human Version of Fenbendazole

Mebendazole is the closest human equivalent to fenbendazole. It's a benzimidazole that treats pinworms, roundworms, hookworms, and whipworms. It's been used in humans for decades. It's safe, cheap, and available over-the-counter in many countries.

2.2.1 The Johns Hopkins Connection

Mebendazole is being studied at Johns Hopkins University for glioblastoma — the most aggressive brain cancer. A Phase 1 clinical trial tested mebendazole in combination with standard chemotherapy (temozolomide) for newly diagnosed glioblastoma.

The rationale: mebendazole crosses the blood-brain barrier (most drugs don't), disrupts tubulin in glioblastoma cells, and has shown activity in preclinical models. If it works, it would be one of the cheapest brain cancer drugs ever developed.

Results from early trials have been promising enough to justify continued investigation. Mebendazole was well-tolerated. Some patients showed extended progression-free survival. Not a cure. But a signal worth pursuing.

2.2.2 Other Cancer Research

Mebendazole has also shown activity in: - Adrenocortical carcinoma - Non-small cell lung cancer - Melanoma - Colon cancer

The research is preclinical. But the consistency across cancer types suggests a real biological mechanism.

Evidence Tier: Moderate preclinical; early clinical (glioblastoma).

2.3 Praziquantel — The Fluke Killer with Indirect Benefits

Praziquantel doesn't directly kill cancer cells. But it removes the parasites that cause cancer — and that makes it one of the most important drugs in this book.

2.3.1 What It Treats

- Schistosoma haematobium (bladder fluke)
- Schistosoma mansoni and japonicum (intestinal flukes)
- Opisthorchis viverrini and Clonorchis sinensis (liver flukes)
- Taenia solium (pork tapeworm — though albendazole is preferred for neurocysticercosis)
- Other flatworm parasites

2.3.2 How It Works

Praziquantel disrupts calcium homeostasis in parasites, causing muscle contraction, tegument (surface membrane) damage, and immune recognition. The parasite is essentially paralyzed and then destroyed by the host immune system.

2.3.3 The Cancer Connection (Indirect)

For patients with proven or suspected parasite-related cancers, praziquantel is essential:

- **Bladder cancer patients with S. haematobium:** Praziquantel removes the carcinogenic stimulus. Without the parasite, the chronic inflammation stops. New lesions may not form. Existing lesions may regress.
- **Cholangiocarcinoma patients with liver flukes:** Praziquantel kills the flukes, stops the bile duct damage, and removes the genotoxic exposure.
- **Post-surgical prevention:** In endemic regions, patients treated for parasite-related cancer should receive praziquantel to prevent recurrence from persistent infection.

Praziquantel also has anti-inflammatory effects that may contribute to a healthier terrain, even in cancers not directly caused by flukes.

Evidence Tier: Proven for parasite removal; indirect for cancer prevention.

2.4 Nitazoxanide — The Forgotten Broad-Spectrum Agent

Nitazoxanide treats protozoan parasites (Giardia, Cryptosporidium) and some helminths. It works by blocking pyruvate:ferredoxin oxidoreductase — an enzyme essential for anaerobic metabolism in parasites.

2.4.1 Emerging Anticancer Research

Nitazoxanide has shown surprising anticancer activity: - **Wnt/β-catenin inhibition:** Blocks a major cancer signaling pathway - **Colorectal cancer:** Reduces proliferation in colon cancer cell lines - **Breast cancer:** Shows anti-proliferative and pro-apoptotic effects - **Prostate cancer:** Inhibits cell growth in prostate cancer models - **Immune modulation:** Enhances antitumor immunity in some models

The Wnt/β-catenin pathway is active in many cancers. Nitazoxanide's ability to inhibit it makes it a broadly interesting candidate. But research is early, and human data is minimal.

Evidence Tier: Emerging preclinical.

2.5 Comparing the Toolkit

Drug	Primary Parasites	Anticancer Mechanism	Human Approval	Clinical Trial Evidence
Ivermectin	Nematodes, ectoparasites	Tubulin, apoptosis, Wnt, P-gp	Yes	None for cancer
Fenbendazole	Veterinary nematodes	Tubulin, glucose, apoptosis	No (veterinary)	None
Albendazole	Echinococcus, nematodes	Tubulin, glucose, apoptosis	Yes	None for cancer
Mebendazole	Nematodes	Tubulin, glucose, apoptosis	Yes	Phase 1 (glioblastoma)
Praziquantel	Flukes, tapeworms	Removes carcinogenic stimulus	Yes	None for cancer
Nitazoxanide	Protozoa, some helminths	Wnt inhibition, immune	Yes	None for cancer

---

2.6 The Combination Strategy

No single drug is likely to be sufficient. The logical approach - based on mechanism, not proven clinical data - is combination:

For parasite-related cancers: - Praziquantel to remove the causative parasite - Albendazole or mebendazole for additional tubulin disruption - Ivermectin for immune modulation - Terrain repair (diet, pH, detox) to prevent recurrence

For non-parasite-related cancers (as adjuncts): - Mebendazole or albendazole for tubulin disruption and metabolic inhibition - Ivermectin for immune modulation and chemosensitization - Nitazoxanide for Wnt pathway inhibition - Conventional treatment as primary therapy

Critical framing: These combinations are theoretical. They're based on mechanism overlap, not clinical trials. Nobody has tested this specific cocktail in humans. Anyone considering combination approaches needs medical supervision, monitoring, and realistic expectations.

2.7 What You Can Do Today

1. If you have a parasite-related cancer, demand treatment for the parasite.

Bladder cancer + schistosomiasis risk → praziquantel. Bile duct cancer + liver fluke risk → praziquantel. This is not alternative medicine. This is standard infectious disease treatment. The fact that oncologists don't think about it doesn't make it optional.

2. Ask your doctor about mebendazole if you have glioblastoma.

Johns Hopkins is studying it. Other centers may be enrolling. If you're eligible for a trial, consider it. Mebendazole is safe, cheap, and crosses the blood-brain barrier — three features that most glioblastoma drugs lack.

3. Don't mix veterinary and human drugs without understanding the difference.

Fenbendazole (veterinary) and mebendazole (human) are similar but not identical. Their pharmacokinetics differ. Their formulations differ. Their safety profiles differ. If you're going to explore benzimidazoles, the human-approved versions (albendazole, mebendazole) are the safer starting point.

4. Look up each drug on PubMed before discussing with your doctor.

Search "albendazole cancer," "mebendazole glioblastoma," "praziquantel schistosomiasis cancer." Print the abstracts. Bring them to your appointment. Your doctor may not know this literature exists.

5. Remember: these drugs treat parasites first.

Even if the anticancer data never pans out, these drugs remove parasites. And removing parasites — especially in cancer patients — is valuable in itself. Parasites suppress immunity, consume nutrients, and create inflammation. Getting rid of them is always a good idea.

Sources & Evidence Tiers for This Chapter:

Claim	Evidence	Tier
Albendazole shows anticancer activity in preclinical models	In vitro studies	**Moderate Preclinical**
Mebendazole in Phase 1 glioblastoma trial at Johns Hopkins	Clinical trial registry	**Early Clinical**
Praziquantel removes carcinogenic flukes	Standard of care for schistosomiasis/flukes	**Established**
Nitazoxanide inhibits Wnt/β-catenin	In vitro studies	**Emerging Preclinical**
Benzimidazoles share tubulin-disruption mechanism	Biochemistry literature	**Established**

Full references with URLs and DOIs are available in Appendix G.

Chapter 17 — Albendazole, Mebendazole, Praziquantel The Parasite-Cancer Connection: What Science Reveals About Hidden Infections, Tumor Mimics, and the Parasites Proven to Cause Cancer

The Parasite-Cancer Connection

What Science Reveals About Hidden Infections, Tumor Mimics, and the Parasites Proven to Cause Cancer

Chapter 18

The Parasite Cleanse Protocol

A Critical Examination

For educational and informational purposes only.
Not medical advice. Consult a qualified healthcare provider.

Table of Contents

1 Chapter 18

2 The Parasite Cleanse Protocol — A Step-by-Step Guide

DISCLAIMER: This chapter is for educational and informational purposes only. It is not medical advice. The protocol described here is a synthesis of practices used by functional medicine practitioners, naturopaths, and integrative oncologists. It has not been validated in randomized controlled trials. Individual needs vary based on cancer type, stage, treatment status, organ function, and overall health. Some components of this protocol may interact with chemotherapy, immunotherapy, or other medications. Always consult a qualified healthcare provider before starting any cleanse, detox, or supplement protocol. This is especially critical for cancer patients, who may have compromised organ function and altered drug metabolism.

By this point in the book, you understand the problem: parasites are linked to cancer, they're routinely missed by standard testing, and they damage the terrain that allows cancer to grow. You also understand the pharmaceutical options: ivermectin, fenbendazole, albendazole, mebendazole, praziquantel, and nitazoxanide.

But drugs alone aren't enough. Parasites don't live in a vacuum. They thrive in acidic, toxic, nutrient-depleted bodies. Kill the parasites without fixing the terrain, and new parasites will move in — or the old ones will survive in cysts, eggs, and dormant stages that drugs don't reach.

This chapter is about the full protocol. Not just killing parasites. Preparing the body to release them. Supporting the organs that process them. Repairing the damage they left behind. And maintaining a terrain that's hostile to reinfection.

2.1 The Principles of Effective Parasite Cleansing

Before the steps, the principles:

1. Drainage before drainage. Your liver, kidneys, colon, and lymphatic system must be able to eliminate parasites and their toxins. If these organs are congested, killing parasites creates a toxic overload — Herxheimer reactions, nausea, headaches, rashes, fatigue. Support elimination organs FIRST.

2. Go slow. Aggressive protocols cause aggressive die-off. Slow protocols cause manageable die-off. The parasites didn't get there overnight. They don't need to leave overnight.

3. Layer the approach. No single drug or herb kills all parasites. Different classes require different treatments. Layer pharmaceutical antiparasitics, herbal antiparasitics, and terrain repair for comprehensive coverage.

4. Test before, during, and after. Baseline testing shows what you're dealing with. Follow-up testing shows whether the protocol worked. Without testing, you're guessing.

5. Individualize. There is no one-size-fits-all protocol. A Stage 4 cancer patient on chemotherapy needs a different approach than a healthy person doing preventive cleansing. Work with a practitioner who can tailor the protocol to your situation.

2.2 Phase 1: Preparation (Week 1-2)

2.2.1 Step 1: Open the Drainage Pathways

Liver support: - Milk thistle (silymarin): 300-600 mg daily, standardized extract - Dandelion root tea: 2-3 cups daily - N-acetyl cysteine (NAC): 600-1200 mg daily (supports glutathione) - Castor oil packs: Apply to liver area (right upper abdomen) for 30-60 minutes, 3-4 times per week

Kidney support: - Hydration: Minimum 2 liters of clean water daily - Parsley tea or extract: Supports kidney filtration - Nettle leaf tea: Gentle kidney support and mineral replacement

Colon support: - Fiber: 30-40 grams daily from vegetables, seeds, and supplemental fiber if needed - Magnesium: 300-500 mg daily (citrate or glycinate)

to ensure daily bowel movements - Probiotics: Multi-strain, high-CFU probiotic to begin rebuilding gut flora

Lymphatic support: - Dry brushing: 5-10 minutes daily before showering - Movement: Walking, rebounding, yoga — anything that moves lymph - Hydration: Essential for lymphatic flow

2.2.2 Step 2: Alkalinize the Terrain

- **Diet shift:** Eliminate sugar, processed foods, alcohol, and factory-farmed meat. Increase leafy greens, vegetables, alkaline fruits (lemons, limes, berries), and clean protein.
- **Morning alkaline drink:** Warm water with juice of half a lemon and 1/4 tsp baking soda (sodium bicarbonate)
- **pH testing:** Monitor urine pH daily. Target: 6.8-7.2 in the morning.

2.2.3 Step 3: Reduce the Toxic Load

- Eliminate alcohol completely during the cleanse
- Eliminate processed foods, preservatives, and artificial sweeteners
- Switch to organic produce to reduce pesticide exposure
- Use natural cleaning products and personal care products
- If you have mercury amalgam fillings, consult a biological dentist (don't remove them during active cancer treatment without specialist guidance)

2.3 Phase 2: Active Parasite Treatment (Weeks 2-6)

2.3.1 Layer 1: Pharmaceutical Antiparasitics

Work with a healthcare provider to determine which drugs are appropriate for your situation. Options include:

Ivermectin: 12-18 mg daily for 5 days, then 2 days off. Repeat for 3-4 cycles. - Consider higher doses (24 mg) only under medical supervision - Take with food to enhance absorption

Albendazole or Mebendazole: 400 mg daily for 3 days, then 4 days off. Repeat for 4-6 cycles. - Albendazole is better absorbed with fatty meals -

Mebendazole can be taken with or without food

Praziquantel: Only if specific fluke or tapeworm infection is suspected or confirmed. - Dose depends on the parasite: typically 40 mg/kg in divided doses for schistosomiasis - Must be prescribed and monitored

Nitazoxanide: 500 mg twice daily for 3 days, for protozoan parasites. - Take with food

Critical: Do NOT combine all these drugs simultaneously without medical supervision. Rotating them or using targeted combinations based on testing is safer and more effective.

2.3.2 Layer 2: Herbal Antiparasitics

Herbs have been used for millennia to treat parasites. They work through different mechanisms than drugs and can target life stages that drugs miss (eggs, cysts, dormant larvae).

Wormwood (Artemisia absinthium): 300-500 mg daily. Contains thujone and other compounds toxic to parasites. Do not use long-term (maximum 4-6 weeks) due to thujone toxicity.

Black walnut hull (Juglans nigra): 500-1000 mg daily. Contains juglone, a compound toxic to parasites and their eggs.

Cloves (Syzygium aromaticum): 500 mg daily or 2-3 whole cloves chewed. The only common herb that reliably targets parasite eggs.

Oregano oil: 150-300 mg daily of standardized extract (minimum 70% carvacrol). Broad-spectrum antimicrobial with antiparasitic properties.

Garlic: 2-4 fresh cloves daily or 600-1200 mg aged garlic extract. Allicin and other sulfur compounds have antiparasitic and immune-enhancing effects.

Papaya seeds: 1 tablespoon daily of ground seeds. Contains carpaine and benzyl isothiocyanate, which have documented antiparasitic effects.

Pumpkin seeds: 1/2 cup daily. Contains cucurbitacin, which paralyzes intestinal worms.

Diatomaceous earth (food grade): 1-2 tablespoons daily in water. Mechanical action damages parasite exoskeletons. Must be food grade (not pool grade). Stay well-hydrated.

2.3.3 Layer 3: Biofilm Disruptors

Parasites and pathogenic bacteria form biofilms — protective slime layers that shield them from drugs and immune attack.

Enzymes: - Serrapeptase or nattokinase: 80,000-120,000 SPU daily, away from meals - These enzymes break down biofilm matrices and expose parasites to treatment

EDTA: Some protocols use EDTA to chelate metals that stabilize biofilms. Use only under supervision.

2.3.4 Layer 4: Bindners (During Die-Off)

When parasites die, they release toxins. Binders capture these toxins in the gut and prevent reabsorption.

Activated charcoal: 500-1000 mg daily, away from medications and supplements (binds to them too)

Bentonite clay: 1 teaspoon in water daily

Chlorella: 2-3 grams daily. Binds toxins and provides nutrients.

Psyllium husk: 1-2 tablespoons daily. Bulks stool and carries toxins out.

Take binders 2 hours away from medications and supplements.

2.4 Phase 3: Recovery and Terrain Repair (Weeks 6-10)

2.4.1 Step 1: Continue Drainage Support

Don't stop liver, kidney, and colon support when the antiparasitics end. The body is still processing dead parasites and repairing damage.

2.4.2 Step 2: Rebuild the Microbiome

Parasites disrupt gut bacteria. Antiparasitic drugs disrupt gut bacteria further. Rebuilding is essential.

Probiotics: Multi-strain, 50-100 billion CFU daily. Include: - Lactobacillus strains (acidophilus, rhamnosus, reuteri) - Bifidobacterium strains (longum, infantis, breve) - Saccharomyces boulardii (beneficial yeast that resists antibiotics)

Prebiotics: Feed beneficial bacteria with: - Inulin and FOS (fructooligosaccharides) - Resistant starch (cooled potatoes, green bananas) - Jerusalem artichoke, chicory root, garlic, onions

Fermented foods: Sauerkraut, kimchi, kefir (if dairy-tolerant), kombucha. Live cultures from food are highly bioavailable.

2.4.3 Step 3: Nutrient Replenishment

Parasites steal nutrients. The cleanse process depletes nutrients. Replenish:

Zinc: 30-50 mg daily (chelated form). Essential for immune function and tissue repair.

Selenium: 200 mcg daily. Critical for thyroid function, antioxidant defense, and immune surveillance.

Vitamin D3: 5,000-10,000 IU daily, based on blood levels. Test 25-OH vitamin D; target 60-80 ng/mL.

Magnesium: Continue 300-500 mg daily. Essential for 300+ enzymatic reactions.

B-complex: Especially B12 and folate, which parasites deplete.

Vitamin C: 2,000-5,000 mg daily in divided doses. Antioxidant and immune support.

Omega-3 fatty acids: 2-3 grams EPA/DHA daily. Anti-inflammatory and membrane repair.

2.4.4 Step 4: Continue Alkalinization

Maintain the alkaline diet. Continue morning alkaline drinks. Monitor pH. The goal is not just to kill parasites but to make the body inhospitable to their return.

2.5 Phase 4: Maintenance (Ongoing)

2.5.1 Monthly or Quarterly Mini-Cleanses

- 3-5 days of herbal antiparasitics (wormwood, black walnut, cloves)
- Probiotic support
- pH monitoring
- Parasite testing every 6-12 months if ongoing risk

2.5.2 Daily Terrain Maintenance

- Alkaline, whole-foods diet
- Clean water (2+ liters daily)
- Regular bowel movements
- Movement and lymphatic support
- Stress management (cortisol suppresses immunity)
- Adequate sleep (immune repair happens during sleep)
- Minimize toxin exposure

2.6 Special Considerations for Cancer Patients

If you're currently undergoing chemotherapy: - Do NOT start parasite cleanses during active chemo without oncologist approval - Some herbs interact with chemotherapy drugs - Die-off reactions may compound chemo side effects - Wait for treatment breaks or work with an integrative oncologist

If you're post-treatment: - This is the ideal time for comprehensive parasite testing and cleansing - Your immune system needs rebuilding - Your gut microbiome has been devastated by treatment - Terrain repair is essential for preventing recurrence

If you're Stage 4 or terminal: - Aggressive parasite treatment may still be valuable — parasites suppress immunity and consume nutrients you desperately need - Focus on tolerable doses and supportive measures - Quality of life matters as much as quantity

If you're a caregiver: - Read this chapter twice - Understand that the protocol must be individualized - Monitor for Herxheimer reactions (die-off symptoms) - Keep a journal of symptoms, doses, and responses

---

2.7 Warning Signs: When to Stop and Seek Help

Stop the cleanse and contact your healthcare provider if you experience: - Severe abdominal pain - Persistent vomiting or diarrhea - Blood in stool or urine - Jaundice (yellowing skin/eyes) - Severe weakness or confusion - Chest pain or difficulty breathing - Signs of allergic reaction (hives, swelling, difficulty breathing)

Mild die-off symptoms are normal: fatigue, headache, body aches, loose stools, skin breakouts. These usually resolve within 3-5 days. Severe symptoms are not normal and require medical attention.

2.8 What You Can Do Today

1. Start with Phase 1 — drainage and alkalinization — before taking any antiparasitic drugs.

Even if you can't get pharmaceutical antiparasitics yet, start the preparation. Open your drainage pathways. Shift your diet. Test your pH. The preparation phase alone will improve how you feel and how you respond to treatment.

2. Order pH test strips and start testing tomorrow morning.

First morning urine, before eating or drinking. Record the number. Do it for 7 days. If you're consistently below 6.5, your terrain needs work.

3. Add one liver-supportive practice this week.

Milk thistle. Dandelion tea. Castor oil pack. Lemon water. Pick one. Do it daily. Your liver processes everything — drugs, toxins, dead parasites. Support it.

4. Read the contraindications for every drug and herb before taking it.

Wormwood is not safe in pregnancy. Black walnut is not safe for people with nut allergies. Activated charcoal binds medications. Know what you're taking and why.

5. Find a practitioner who understands this work.

A functional medicine doctor. A naturopathic oncologist. An integrative MD. Someone who can supervise the protocol, order tests, adjust doses, and manage side effects. Don't do this alone.

Sources & Evidence Tiers for This Chapter:

Claim	Evidence	Tier
Milk thistle supports liver function	Multiple clinical studies	**Established**
Magnesium supports bowel regularity	Clinical nutrition literature	**Established**
Probiotics restore gut microbiome after treatment	Meta-analyses	**Established**
Wormwood, black walnut, cloves have antiparasitic properties	Traditional use + modern pharmacology	**Traditional/ Moderate**
Biofilms protect parasites from treatment	Microbiology literature	**Established**
pH affects parasite survival	Biological plausibility	**Plausible**
Die-off (Herxheimer) reactions occur with parasite killing	Clinical observations	**Established**
This specific protocol has not been validated in RCTs	Absence of trials	**Not Proven**

Full references with URLs and DOIs are available in Appendix G.

Chapter 18 — The Parasite Cleanse Protocol The Parasite-Cancer Connection: What Science Reveals About Hidden Infections, Tumor Mimics, and the Parasites Proven to Cause Cancer

The Parasite-Cancer Connection

What Science Reveals About Hidden Infections, Tumor Mimics, and the Parasites Proven to Cause Cancer

Chapter 19

pH, Diet, and Terrain Repair

A Critical Examination

For educational and informational purposes only.
Not medical advice. Consult a qualified healthcare provider.

Table of Contents

1 Chapter 19

2 pH, Diet, and Terrain Repair — Rebuilding the Soil

DISCLAIMER: This chapter is for educational and informational purposes only. It is not medical advice. The dietary and lifestyle recommendations described here are based on nutritional science, epidemiological studies, and integrative medicine practice. Individual needs vary based on cancer type, treatment status, organ function, metabolic state, and food sensitivities. Some dietary changes may interact with medications or treatments. Cancer patients with compromised organ function, cachexia, or specific metabolic restrictions should work with a registered dietitian or physician before making major dietary changes. Always consult a qualified healthcare provider before making any health decisions.

We've talked about killing parasites. We've talked about drugs. Now we need to talk about the foundation: the terrain. The internal environment. The soil in which disease grows or withers.

If you kill every parasite in your body but leave the terrain acidic, toxic, and depleted, new parasites will arrive within weeks. Cancer cells will find the same hospitable environment. The cycle continues.

This chapter is about fixing the soil. pH. Diet. Detoxification. The things that don't come in a pill but determine whether any pill works.

2.1 pH — The Acidity-Cancer-Parasite Triangle

Your blood maintains a tight pH range: 7.35-7.45. Deviate outside this range, and you die. Your body will sacrifice bone mineral density, muscle mass, and organ function to keep blood pH stable.

But your tissues — the spaces between cells — can become acidic without killing you. Your urine pH can drop below 6.0. Your saliva pH can be acidic. Your intracellular pH shifts in disease states. And in these compartments, acidity matters enormously.

2.1.1 Why Cancer Loves Acid

Cancer cells produce lactic acid through glycolysis (the Warburg effect). This acidifies the tumor microenvironment. But the acidity is not just a byproduct — it's a weapon:

- **Acid promotes angiogenesis:** Tumors need blood vessels. Acidic pH stimulates VEGF (vascular endothelial growth factor), which builds new vessels to feed the tumor.
- **Acid promotes metastasis:** Cancer cells in acidic environments become more invasive. The acid breaks down surrounding tissue, creating pathways for escape.
- **Acid suppresses immunity:** Immune cells function poorly in acidic environments. Natural killer cells, T cells, and macrophages all lose effectiveness below pH 7.0.
- **Acid promotes drug resistance:** Many chemotherapy drugs become less effective in acidic environments. The tumor creates its own shield.

2.1.2 Why Parasites Love Acid

Parasites also prefer acidic environments: - **Toxoplasma gondii** thrives in acidic vacuoles within host cells - **Trichomonas vaginalis** lives in the acidic vaginal environment - **Helicobacter pylori** (the bacterium that causes ulcers and stomach cancer) survives by neutralizing stomach acid — but it needs the acidic environment to activate its virulence factors - **Echinococcus** cysts maintain an acidic internal environment that suppresses immune attack

When the body is acidic, parasites find a home. When parasites establish, they create more acidity. The cycle feeds itself.

2.1.3 How to Measure and Change pH

Testing: - **Urine pH:** Test first morning urine with pH strips. Healthy range: 6.5-7.5. Below 6.0 = too acidic. - **Saliva pH:** Test before eating or drinking.

Healthy range: 6.5-7.5. - **Track trends:** One test doesn't matter. Track for 2 weeks to see your pattern.

Alkalinization strategies: - **Diet:** See below. This is the primary tool. - **Baking soda (sodium bicarbonate):** 1/4 to 1/2 teaspoon in water, 1-2 times daily. Cheap, effective, but use cautiously if you have high blood pressure, kidney disease, or are on sodium-restricted diets. - **Potassium bicarbonate:** Alternative for those who need to limit sodium. - **Magnesium:** Supports alkalinization and is essential for 300+ reactions. - **Deep breathing:** CO2 retention acidifies blood. Slow, deep breathing alkalinizes.

Important: Don't over-alkalinize. Extreme alkalosis (pH > 7.5 in blood) is dangerous. Target tissue pH improvement, not blood pH manipulation. Work with a practitioner if you're uncertain.

2.2 Diet — The Single Most Powerful Terrain Tool

You eat 3-5 times a day. Every meal is a message to your body. Every bite either builds health or depletes it. There is no neutral food.

2.2.1 What to Eliminate

Sugar and refined carbohydrates: Cancer cells consume glucose at 10-20x the rate of normal cells. Sugar is their primary fuel. Eliminating sugar doesn't starve cancer entirely (the body makes glucose from other sources), but it reduces the excess fuel that drives proliferation. Parasites also thrive on sugar. Starve them both.

Factory-farmed meat and dairy: These contain hormones, antibiotics, pesticide residues, and inflammatory omega-6 fats. They also contribute to acidity. If you eat animal products, choose grass-fed, organic, pasture-raised.

Processed foods: Preservatives, artificial colors, flavorings, and trans fats all add to the toxic load. The body processes them as foreign substances, diverting energy from repair to detoxification.

Alcohol: A Group 1 carcinogen according to IARC. Damages the liver, depletes nutrients, disrupts sleep, and feeds parasites and yeast.

Industrial seed oils: Soybean oil, corn oil, canola oil, sunflower oil — these are high in omega-6 fatty acids that promote inflammation. Use olive oil, coconut oil, avocado oil, or butter from grass-fed cows instead.

2.2.2 What to Emphasize

Leafy greens and vegetables: The most alkaline foods. Kale, spinach, collards, Swiss chard, arugula, romaine, bok choy. Aim for 6-9 cups daily. Yes, cups. This is the foundation.

Cruciferous vegetables: Broccoli, cauliflower, Brussels sprouts, cabbage, kohlrabi. These contain sulforaphane and indole-3-carbinol — compounds that support liver detoxification, hormone balance, and immune function.

Alkaline fruits: Lemons, limes, grapefruits, berries, melons. Despite their acidic taste, these alkalinize the body. (Lemon water in the morning is a classic alkalinizing practice.)

Clean protein: Wild-caught fish (salmon, sardines, mackerel), pasture-raised poultry, grass-fed beef, organic eggs, legumes, and properly prepared plant proteins.

Healthy fats: Avocado, olive oil, coconut oil, nuts, seeds, and fatty fish. These support hormone production, cell membrane integrity, and anti-inflammatory signaling.

Fermented foods: Sauerkraut, kimchi, kefir, kombucha. These introduce beneficial bacteria and support the gut microbiome — which, as we established in Chapter 11, is central to immune function and cancer resistance.

Filtered water: Chlorine and fluoride in tap water disrupt gut bacteria and thyroid function. Use a quality water filter (reverse osmosis or carbon block with fluoride removal).

2.2.3 The 80/20 Alkaline Rule

You don't need to be perfect. Aim for 80% alkaline-forming foods and 20% acid-forming foods. This creates a net alkaline effect without making you crazy.

Track your meals for 3 days. Count alkaline vs. acid foods. Most people eating a standard Western diet are at 20/80 — the inverse of what creates health.

2.3 Detoxification — Reducing the Toxic Load

Your body has detoxification systems: liver (phase 1 and 2 enzymes), kidneys (filtration), colon (elimination), lungs (volatile compounds), skin (sweating), and lymphatic system (drainage). These systems can be overwhelmed by modern toxic exposure.

2.3.1 Sources of Toxic Load

Environmental: Air pollution, industrial chemicals, pesticides, herbicides, heavy metals, plastics (BPA, phthalates), flame retardants, forever chemicals (PFAS).

Food: Pesticide residues, preservatives, artificial sweeteners, food dyes, packaging chemicals.

Water: Chlorine, fluoride, pharmaceutical residues, agricultural runoff.

Products: Commercial cleaning products, air fresheners, cosmetics, personal care products with parabens, sulfates, and synthetic fragrances.

Dental: Mercury amalgam fillings, root canal infections.

Medical: Chemotherapy drugs, radiation, diagnostic contrast agents, antibiotics.

2.3.2 Detox Support Strategies

Liver Phase 1 support: - B-vitamins (especially B6, B12, folate) - Antioxidants (vitamin C, vitamin E, selenium, glutathione) - Cruciferous vegetables

Liver Phase 2 support (conjugation): - Glutathione (NAC, glycine, glutamine support production) - Sulfur-rich foods (garlic, onions, eggs, cruciferous vegetables) - Amino acids (taurine, glycine, methionine) - Molybdenum (supports sulfite oxidase)

Kidney support: - Hydration (2+ liters clean water daily) - Nettle leaf, parsley, dandelion - Low-sodium diet if kidney function is compromised

Colon support: - Fiber (30-40 grams daily) - Regular bowel movements (daily elimination is essential for detox) - Probiotics and fermented foods

Skin support: - Sweating: sauna, exercise, hot baths - Dry brushing to stimulate lymphatic drainage

Lymphatic support: - Movement (walking, rebounding, yoga) - Deep breathing - Lymphatic massage

2.3.3 Special Considerations for Cancer Patients

During chemotherapy: - Focus on gentle detox support. Avoid aggressive protocols that may interfere with drug metabolism. - Hydration is paramount. - Liver support (milk thistle, NAC) may help protect against chemo-induced liver damage — discuss with your oncologist.

During radiation: - Antioxidants are controversial during radiation (theoretically, they might protect cancer cells from radiation damage). Some oncologists restrict antioxidants during radiation. Others allow them. Ask your radiation oncologist.

Post-treatment: - This is when aggressive detox makes sense. Your body has been through chemical warfare. It needs support to clear residual toxins. - Consider working with an integrative practitioner on a comprehensive detox protocol.

2.4 Sleep, Stress, and Movement — The Non-Nutritional Terrain Factors

Sleep: During sleep, the body repairs DNA, clears metabolic waste through the glymphatic system, replenishes neurotransmitters, and restores immune function. Chronic sleep deprivation increases inflammation, suppresses immunity, and promotes cancer progression. Target 7-9 hours. Quality matters as much as quantity — deep sleep and REM sleep are essential.

Stress: Chronic stress elevates cortisol, which suppresses immune surveillance, promotes inflammation, and drives insulin resistance. Stress also acidifies the body and disrupts sleep. Stress management is not a luxury — it's a biological necessity. Meditation, breathing exercises, nature exposure, social connection, and creative activities all reduce cortisol and improve terrain.

Movement: Exercise improves lymphatic drainage, oxygenates tissues, reduces inflammation, balances hormones, and supports mood. But extreme exercise (marathons, ultra-endurance) creates oxidative stress and immune suppression. Moderate, consistent movement — walking, swimming, yoga, strength training — is ideal. Listen to your body. Rest when needed.

2.5 What You Can Do Today

1. Test your pH tomorrow morning.

Buy pH strips. Test first morning urine. Record the number. If it's below 6.5, start the alkalinization strategies in this chapter.

2. Make one dietary swap this week.

Replace one acid-forming food with one alkaline-forming food. Sugar-sweetened beverage → lemon water. Factory-farmed meat → wild-caught fish. Processed snack → raw vegetables with hummus. One swap. This week.

3. Increase your vegetable intake by one cup today.

Most people eat 1-2 cups of vegetables daily. The target is 6-9. Add one cup today. A salad. A green smoothie. Steamed broccoli with dinner. One cup. Build from there.

4. Audit your home for toxin sources.

Walk through your house. Look at cleaning products, personal care products, air fresheners, plastic containers, non-stick cookware. Replace one toxic product with a natural alternative this month. Castile soap instead of antibacterial soap. Stainless steel instead of Teflon. Glass instead of plastic for food storage.

5. Prioritize sleep tonight.

Set a bedtime. Turn off screens 1 hour before. Darken the room. Cool the temperature. Sleep is when your body repairs. Nothing else you do matters if you're not sleeping.

Sources & Evidence Tiers for This Chapter:

Claim	Evidence	Tier
Cancer thrives in acidic microenvironments	Tumor microenvironment literature	**Established**
Acidic pH promotes angiogenesis and metastasis	Cancer biology literature	**Established**
Diet affects body pH and inflammation	Nutritional epidemiology	**Established**
Sugar feeds cancer cells (Warburg effect)	Biochemistry; Otto Warburg	**Established**
Cruciferous vegetables support detoxification	Nutritional science	**Established**
Sleep deprivation impairs immunity	Sleep medicine literature	**Established**
Chronic stress elevates cortisol and suppresses immunity	Psychoneuroimmunology	**Established**
Processed foods increase toxic load	Environmental health literature	**Established**

Full references with URLs and DOIs are available in Appendix G.

The Parasite-Cancer Connection

What Science Reveals About Hidden Infections, Tumor Mimics, and the Parasites Proven to Cause Cancer

Chapter 20

Building Your Second Look Team

A Critical Examination

For educational and informational purposes only.
Not medical advice. Consult a qualified healthcare provider.

Table of Contents

1 Chapter 20

2 Building Your Second Look Team — Who You Need in Your Corner

---

DISCLAIMER: This chapter is for educational and informational purposes only. It is not medical advice. The practitioners described here have different training, credentials, and scopes of practice. Some are MDs with conventional medical licenses. Others are naturopaths, functional medicine practitioners, or integrative health coaches. The choice of practitioners is a personal decision that should be based on your health status, treatment goals, and comfort level. Always verify credentials, check for disciplinary actions, and interview any practitioner before engaging their services. This chapter does not endorse any specific practitioner or approach.

You can't do this alone. Cancer is too complex. Parasites are too hidden. The medical system is too stacked against you. You need a team — a group of people who see what you see, who ask the questions you're asking, and who have the skills to help you find answers.

This chapter is about building that team. Not just any team. Your team. The people who will look where others won't look, test what others won't test, and treat what others won't treat.

2.1 The Core Team Members

2.1.1 1. The Conventional Oncologist (Yes, You Still Need One)

I know this book is critical of oncology. But the truth is: conventional oncology has tools that save lives. Surgery removes tumors. Radiation kills localized cancer. Chemotherapy works for some cancers. Immunotherapy is transformative for some patients. Targeted therapy offers precision that wasn't possible a decade ago.

The oncologist's role on your team is: - Diagnosis and staging - Conventional treatment planning - Monitoring tumor markers and imaging - Managing acute complications - Providing emergency care

The key is finding an oncologist who: - Respects your questions and autonomy - Doesn't dismiss alternative approaches out of hand - Is willing to collaborate with other practitioners - Explains risks and benefits honestly - Doesn't pressure you into immediate decisions

Red flags: - "We need to start treatment tomorrow" (without adequate explanation) - "Don't waste your time with that stuff" (dismissive of all alternatives) - "This is the only option" (when second opinions exist) - Refuses to discuss side effects or prognosis - Makes you feel stupid for asking questions

Green flags: - "Let's talk through all your options" - "I don't know much about that, but I'm open to learning" - "Here are the risks and benefits. The decision is yours." - Refers you to integrative colleagues - Respects your timeline for decision-making

2.1.2 2. The Integrative or Functional Medicine Doctor

This is your second-look quarterback. The person who asks "why" instead of "what." The person who runs comprehensive testing, looks for root causes, and builds protocols that address the whole person.

Credentials to look for: - MD or DO with additional training in integrative or functional medicine - Certified by the Institute for Functional Medicine (IFM) - Member of the Integrative Oncology association - Naturopathic oncologist (ND with oncology specialization)

What they do: - Comprehensive gut testing (stool PCR, not just basic O&P) - Food sensitivity and allergy testing - Heavy metal and mold testing - Hormone panels - Nutrient status testing - pH and metabolic testing - Parasite testing (comprehensive panels) - Terrain-repair protocols (diet, supplements, lifestyle) - Adjunct therapies (vitamin C, mistletoe, hyperthermia, etc.)

Interview questions: - "How do you approach parasite testing in cancer patients?" - "What is your experience with antiparasitic drugs as adjuncts?" - "How do you coordinate care with conventional oncologists?" - "What is your philosophy on terrain repair?" - "Can you walk me through a typical protocol?"

2.1.3 3. The Infectious Disease Specialist

If parasites are on your radar, you need someone who actually knows parasites. Most oncologists don't. Most primary care doctors don't. Infectious disease (ID) specialists do.

When to involve an ID specialist: - Positive or suspicious parasite tests - Travel history to endemic regions - Symptoms suggestive of parasitic infection - Need for antiparasitic drug prescriptions (praziquantel, albendazole) - Complex or resistant infections

What they do: - Interpret serology and PCR results - Prescribe appropriate antiparasitic medications - Monitor for drug interactions and side effects - Manage complicated or disseminated infections - Coordinate with oncology for timing of treatment

Finding one: - University hospitals often have tropical medicine specialists - Travel medicine clinics - Major medical centers in urban areas - Ask your oncologist for a referral

2.1.4 4. The Nutrition Professional

Food is medicine. But not generic food advice — "eat healthy" is useless. You need targeted nutritional therapy based on your cancer type, treatment status, lab results, and metabolic state.

Credentials: - Registered Dietitian (RD) with oncology certification (CSO) - Certified Nutrition Specialist (CNS) - Functional medicine nutritionist - Integrative nutrition health coach

What they do: - Assess nutritional status and deficiencies - Design cancer-specific meal plans - Manage treatment side effects through diet (nausea, mouth sores, taste changes) - Support immune function through nutrition - Adjust protocols based on lab work and symptoms - Monitor weight, muscle mass, and metabolic markers

Critical for cancer patients: Malnutrition is common in cancer and worsens outcomes. A good nutrition professional prevents cachexia (muscle wasting), maintains strength, and supports treatment tolerance.

2.1.5 5. The Mental Health Professional

Cancer is not just physical. It's emotional, psychological, existential. Depression, anxiety, trauma, and grief are normal responses to abnormal circumstances. You need someone to help you process them.

Options: - Oncology social worker - Psychologist or psychiatrist with cancer experience - Counselor or therapist - Support group facilitator - Mind-body practitioner (hypnotherapist, meditation teacher)

What they do: - Help process diagnosis, prognosis, and treatment decisions - Manage treatment-related anxiety and depression - Support family communication - Address existential questions (meaning, mortality, purpose) - Teach coping skills (mindfulness, CBT, ACT) - Provide a safe space to express fear, anger, and grief

Don't skip this. Mental health affects immune function, treatment adherence, pain perception, and quality of life. It's not a luxury. It's part of the protocol.

2.1.6 6. The Caregiver Advocate

You need someone who is not you. Someone who can: - Attend appointments and take notes - Ask questions you forget to ask - Research treatment options - Coordinate between practitioners - Manage medications and schedules - Provide emotional support - Make calls and handle logistics - Be your voice when you can't speak

This might be a spouse, partner, parent, adult child, sibling, or close friend. It might be a professional patient advocate. Whoever it is, choose someone who: - Has time and availability - Can handle medical information without panicking - Respects your decisions even when they disagree - Communicates clearly with doctors - Is organized and detail-oriented

---

2.2 How to Coordinate Your Team

Having multiple practitioners is powerful — if they communicate. If they don't, you get conflicting advice, duplicated tests, and dangerous drug interactions.

2.2.1 The Medical Binder

Create a physical or digital binder containing: - Diagnosis and pathology reports - Imaging reports (CT, MRI, PET, ultrasound) - Blood work and lab results - Genetic testing results - Treatment history (dates, drugs, doses, responses) - Current medications and supplements (with doses) - Allergies and sensitivities - Contact information for all team members - Appointment notes and questions

Bring this binder to every appointment. Give copies to key team members. Update it regularly.

2.2.2 The Care Coordination Call

Once a month (or after major decisions), have a call or meeting with your primary practitioners — oncologist, integrative doctor, and ID specialist — to: - Share updates - Align on next steps - Resolve conflicts - Adjust protocols - Ensure no dangerous interactions

Not all practitioners will participate. Some are too busy. Some are territorial. But if you can get even two of them talking, you reduce errors and improve care.

2.2.3 The Timeline

Create a written timeline of your care: - Date of diagnosis - Dates of surgeries, biopsies, scans - Dates of treatments (chemo cycles, radiation sessions) - Dates of tests and results - Dates of significant symptoms or side effects - Dates of protocol changes

This timeline helps every new practitioner understand your history quickly. It prevents you from retelling your story endlessly. And it reveals patterns that might otherwise be missed.

2.3 Financial Considerations

Integrative and functional medicine is often not covered by insurance. This creates a cruel reality: the most comprehensive care is the least affordable.

Strategies to manage costs:

Prioritize testing: Spend money on the tests that guide treatment, not on every possible test. A comprehensive stool PCR panel ($200-400) is more valuable than a $2,000 "full body scan" for parasite purposes.

Use insurance when possible: - Conventional testing (blood work, imaging) is usually covered - Some insurance plans cover naturopathic or integrative practitioners - Health savings accounts (HSAs) and flexible spending accounts (FSAs) can be used for many out-of-pocket costs - Some supplements are FSA/HSA eligible

Be strategic about supplements: - Don't buy everything at once - Start with the highest-priority nutrients based on testing - Use quality brands but avoid overpriced boutique products - Buy in bulk when appropriate

Seek community resources: - Cancer support organizations sometimes fund integrative care - Clinical trials may provide free testing and treatment - Some integrative practitioners offer sliding-scale fees - University hospitals sometimes have lower-cost integrative clinics

Track every expense: Medical expenses are tax-deductible above a certain threshold. Keep receipts for: - Practitioner fees - Testing - Supplements and medications - Travel to medical appointments - Medical equipment and supplies

---

2.4 What You Can Do Today

1. Write down your current team.

List every practitioner you're currently seeing: oncologist, primary care, surgeon, radiologist, nutritionist, therapist, etc. Next to each name, write: What do they do for me? Are they open to collaboration? Do I trust them?

2. Identify the gaps.

Do you have an integrative or functional medicine practitioner? Do you have someone who tests for root causes? Do you have a nutrition professional? Do you have mental health support? Do you have a caregiver advocate? Whatever's missing is your next priority.

3. Research one new practitioner this week.

Search the IFM directory, integrative oncology associations, or naturopathic oncology organizations. Find one practitioner in your area. Read their website. Check their reviews. Call their office. Ask about a consultation.

4. Start your medical binder today.

Gather your existing records. Create a folder — physical or digital. Organize by category: diagnosis, imaging, labs, treatments, supplements, appointments. You don't need to finish it today. Just start.

5. Ask your current oncologist one collaboration question.

"Would you be open to communicating with an integrative practitioner if I added one to my team?" Their answer tells you everything about whether they're a team player or a solo act.

Sources & Evidence Tiers for This Chapter:

Claim	Evidence	Tier
Multidisciplinary care improves cancer outcomes	Oncology care coordination literature	**Established**
Integrative medicine addresses root causes	Integrative medicine literature	**Established approach**
Malnutrition worsens cancer outcomes	Clinical nutrition literature	**Established**
Mental health affects immune function	Psychoneuroimmunology	**Established**
Caregiver support improves patient outcomes	Oncology support literature	**Established**
Financial barriers limit access to integrative care	Healthcare economics literature	**Established**

Full references with URLs and DOIs are available in Appendix G.

Chapter 20 — Building Your Second Look Team The Parasite-Cancer Connection: What Science Reveals About Hidden Infections, Tumor Mimics, and the Parasites Proven to Cause Cancer

The Parasite-Cancer Connection

What Science Reveals About Hidden Infections, Tumor Mimics, and the Parasites Proven to Cause Cancer

Chapter 21

How to Talk to Your Doctor About Parasites

A Critical Examination

For educational and informational purposes only.
Not medical advice. Consult a qualified healthcare provider.

Table of Contents

1 Chapter 21

2 How to Talk to Your Doctor About Parasites

DISCLAIMER: This chapter is for educational and informational purposes only. It is not medical advice. The communication strategies described here are designed to help patients have productive conversations with healthcare providers. They do not guarantee that doctors will agree with your perspective, order tests you request, or prescribe treatments you suggest. The goal is respectful, evidence-based dialogue — not adversarial confrontation. Some doctors will be receptive; others will not. This chapter prepares you for both outcomes. Always consult a qualified healthcare provider before making any health decisions.

You've read the book. You've seen the evidence. You want parasite testing. You want a second look. You want your doctor to take this seriously.

And you're terrified that they'll laugh at you.

This chapter is about having that conversation without getting dismissed, without burning bridges, and without being labeled a difficult patient. It's about being heard, not humored.

2.1 Why Doctors Dismiss the Parasite Question

Before the conversation, understand the resistance. Doctors don't dismiss parasites because they're cruel or closed-minded. They dismiss them because:

1. Training: Medical education barely covers parasitology in developed countries. Most doctors see parasites as "tropical diseases" that don't affect their patients.

2. Epidemiology: In their clinical experience, parasites are rare. They see cancer every day. They see parasites once a year, if ever. The base rate affects their judgment.

3. Time pressure: A standard oncology appointment is 15-20 minutes. Parasite discussion takes time the doctor doesn't have.

4. Cognitive dissonance: If parasites are a significant cancer cause, doctors have been missing them for years. That's uncomfortable to admit. It's easier to dismiss the idea.

5. Systemic bias: The medical system rewards cancer diagnosis and treatment, not parasite testing. Doctors are trained in what the system values.

6. Fear of liability: Ordering unusual tests or prescribing off-label drugs creates medicolegal risk. Doctors are trained to minimize risk.

Understanding this doesn't make the dismissal acceptable. But it helps you approach the conversation strategically, not emotionally.

2.2 The Preparation Phase

2.2.1 Step 1: Know Your Evidence

Don't walk in with "I read a book." Walk in with specific, citable research:

- The IARC Monographs classifying S. haematobium and O. viverrini as Group 1 carcinogens
- The 2025 meta-analysis showing 28.42% parasite prevalence in cancer patients
- The NEJM case of Hymenolepis nana becoming cancerous
- The specific studies linking your cancer type to specific parasites (from Chapter 7)
- The CDC's own guidance on false-negative testing (from Chapter 8)

Print abstracts. Highlight key sentences. Bring them with you.

2.2.2 Step 2: Know Your Risk Factors

Document any risk factors for parasitic infection: - Travel history (countries, dates, activities) - Dietary history (raw fish, undercooked meat, unwashed produce) - Animal exposure (pets, livestock, veterinary work) - Water exposure (swimming, freshwater activities) - Prior diagnoses of parasitic infection - Symptoms suggestive of parasites (diarrhea, abdominal pain, unexplained weight loss, itching, rashes) - Immune status (steroid use, chemotherapy, HIV, transplant)

2.2.3 Step 3: Know What Tests You Want

Be specific. Don't say "test me for parasites." Say:

- "I'd like a comprehensive stool PCR panel that includes Blastocystis, Cryptosporidium, Giardia, Dientamoeba, and helminth DNA detection."
- "I'd like serology for Echinococcus, Strongyloides, Toxoplasma, and schistosomiasis."
- "Given my travel history to [country], I'd like liver fluke testing."
- "Given my urinary symptoms and bladder cancer diagnosis, I'd like schistosomiasis testing."

Specific requests are harder to dismiss than vague ones.

2.2.4 Step 4: Know Your Doctor's Style

Some doctors respond to: - **Evidence:** "Here are three peer-reviewed studies." - **Emotion:** "I'm terrified that something is being missed." - **Pragmatism:** "The test is cheap, non-invasive, and has no downside." - **Authority:** "My integrative doctor recommended this." - **Logic:** "If parasites cause cancer in some populations, and I have risk factors, doesn't it make sense to rule it out?"

Figure out which approach resonates with your doctor. Use it.

2.3 The Conversation Script

Here's a framework for the conversation. Adapt it to your style and your doctor's personality.

2.3.1 Opening: Frame the Request

"I've been researching factors that might be contributing to my [cancer type]. I came across some studies linking specific parasites to this cancer. I know it's not mainstream, but I'd like to rule it out. Can we discuss testing?"

This opening: - Acknowledges that you know it's non-mainstream (reduces defensiveness) - Frames it as "ruling out" rather than "proving" (less threatening) - Asks permission to discuss (respectful)

2.3.2 Present the Evidence

"I've printed some abstracts. The IARC classifies Schistosoma haematobium as a Group 1 carcinogen for bladder cancer. [Or: The IARC classifies Opisthorchis viverrini as a Group 1 carcinogen for bile duct cancer.] A 2025 meta-analysis found that 28% of cancer patients harbor parasites. Given my [travel history / symptoms / risk factors], I think testing is warranted."

Hand over the abstracts. Let the doctor read them. Silence is okay — let them process.

2.3.3 Address the Likely Objections

Objection: "You don't have risk factors." Response: "Risk factors are often unknown. I've traveled to [country] / eaten [food] / had [exposure] years ago. Parasites can live for decades. And the meta-analysis shows that even without obvious risk factors, cancer patients have high parasite prevalence. Can we test to be sure?"

Objection: "Your stool test was negative." Response: "I understand that one basic O&P test has limitations. The CDC says multiple tests may be needed for some parasites. I'd like a comprehensive PCR panel and serology to be thorough. Can we order those?"

Objection: "There's no evidence parasites cause [your cancer]." Response: "I understand the evidence is stronger for some cancers than others. For [my cancer], the link is [emerging / speculative / nonexistent]. But parasites suppress immunity and create inflammation, which contributes to all cancers. And I have symptoms that suggest infection. Can we test to rule it out as a contributing factor?"

Objection: "This isn't standard of care." Response: "I understand. But standard of care evolves based on new evidence. The IARC classifications are standard of care for the parasites they cover. For me, the question is whether I have one of those parasites. The test is simple. The downside is minimal. I'd like to proceed."

Objection: "I don't believe in alternative medicine." Response: "This isn't alternative medicine. These are WHO and IARC classifications. These are CDC testing guidelines. This is mainstream parasitology applied to oncology. The only 'alternative' part is that most oncologists don't think to ask the question."

2.3.4 Close with a Specific Request

"Can we order [specific test] today? I'd like to get the results before my next treatment decision."

Be specific. Be time-bound. Make it easy for the doctor to say yes.

2.4 If the Doctor Says No

You did everything right. You brought evidence. You were respectful. You made a reasonable request. And the doctor still said no.

Now what?

2.4.1 Option 1: Ask for Documentation

"I understand you don't think testing is indicated. Can you document in my chart that I requested [specific test] and you declined, including your reasoning?"

This creates a paper trail. It shows you're serious. And it gives the doctor a moment to reconsider — because declining a reasonable request in writing feels different than declining verbally.

2.4.2 Option 2: Ask for a Referral

"If you don't think testing is warranted, can you refer me to an infectious disease specialist or a doctor who might have a different perspective?"

This shifts the decision to another qualified professional. It doesn't force the oncologist to order tests they don't want to order. But it keeps the process moving.

2.4.3 Option 3: Seek a Second Opinion

Find another oncologist. Find an integrative medicine doctor. Find an infectious disease specialist. Find a naturopathic oncologist. Someone, somewhere, will listen.

How to frame the second opinion: "I'd like a second opinion on whether parasite testing is indicated given my risk factors and cancer type. Can you recommend someone, or should I find someone independently?"

2.4.4 Option 4: Order the Test Yourself

In some jurisdictions, patients can order their own laboratory tests through direct-to-consumer labs. Stool PCR panels, serology, and other parasite tests are available without a doctor's order in many areas.

Pros: You get the data. No doctor gatekeeping. **Cons:** Insurance won't cover it. You'll pay out of pocket ($200-500). You'll need someone to interpret results.

If you go this route: - Use a reputable lab - Order a comprehensive panel, not a single test - Bring the results to EVERY practitioner on your team - Don't try to self-treat based on results — get professional interpretation

2.4.5 Option 5: Accept the No and Move On

Sometimes, despite your best effort, the answer is no. The doctor won't test. The system won't budge. The gate is closed.

At that point, you have a choice: fight the system, or work around it. Fighting takes energy you may not have. Working around it — through direct-to-consumer testing, integrative practitioners, or self-advocacy — may be more practical.

You are not required to accept every "no." You are the owner of your body. The doctor is a consultant. The final decision is yours.

2.5 Special Scenarios

2.5.1 Talking to Your Oncologist About Antiparasitics

This is harder than asking for testing. Most oncologists will not prescribe ivermectin, fenbendazole, or mebendazole for cancer.

Frame it as adjunct, not replacement: "I'm not suggesting we stop chemotherapy. I'm asking whether we could add [specific drug] as an adjunct, given the preclinical data on [specific mechanism]. Can we discuss whether this might be compatible with my current regimen?"

Bring the research: Print the specific studies. Not internet articles — PubMed abstracts. Show that the request is evidence-based, not whimsical.

Acknowledge the limitations: "I know the human data is limited. I know this is off-label. I'm not expecting a cure. I'm exploring whether this might help my immune system or reduce inflammation alongside standard treatment."

If they say no: "I understand. Can you document your reasoning? And can you refer me to an integrative oncologist who might be willing to discuss this?"

2.5.2 Talking to Family About Your Choices

Your family may not understand why you're asking about parasites instead of just doing what the oncologist says. They may be scared, skeptical, or angry.

Frame it as thoroughness, not rejection: "I'm not rejecting conventional treatment. I'm making sure we haven't missed anything. The testing is cheap and harmless. If it's negative, we move forward with confidence. If it's positive, we have more information."

Share the evidence: Show them the IARC classifications. Show them the CDC testing guidance. Show them the NEJM case. When family sees that this is real science, not internet quackery, they often become supportive.

Set boundaries: "I appreciate your concern. I've made my decision. I need your support, not your opposition. If you can't support this, please don't argue with me about it."

2.6 What You Can Do Today

1. Print three abstracts from this book and put them in your medical file.

The IARC Group 1 classification abstract. The 2025 meta-analysis abstract. The CDC false-negative testing guidance. These are your evidence foundation.

2. Write down your risk factors in one document.

Travel, diet, exposure, symptoms. Everything that makes parasite testing reasonable for YOU. Personalize the evidence.

3. Practice the opening sentence.

"I've been researching factors that might be contributing to my cancer, and I'd like to discuss some testing that I think is warranted." Say it out loud. Five times. Until it sounds natural.

4. Identify your doctor's likely objections and write responses.

What will they say? "You don't have risk factors." "Your tests were negative." "This isn't standard of care." Write your response to each. Be ready.

5. Schedule the conversation.

Don't bring this up at the end of an appointment when the doctor is rushing out. Schedule a dedicated appointment — or a phone call — to discuss this specifically. Give it the time it deserves.

Sources & Evidence Tiers for This Chapter:

Claim	Evidence	Tier
Doctors receive minimal parasitology training in developed countries	Medical education surveys	**Established**
IARC classifications are mainstream science	IARC Monographs	**Established**

Claim	Evidence	Tier
Patients can order direct-to-consumer lab tests	Direct-to-consumer testing industry	**Established**
Specific, evidence-based requests are harder to dismiss	Communication psychology	**Established**
Second opinions improve diagnostic accuracy	Medical error literature	**Established**

Full references with URLs and DOIs are available in Appendix G.

The Parasite-Cancer Connection

What Science Reveals About Hidden Infections, Tumor Mimics, and the Parasites Proven to Cause Cancer

Chapter 22

Your Action Plan — The 30-Day Challenge

A Critical Examination

For educational and informational purposes only.
Not medical advice. Consult a qualified healthcare provider.

Table of Contents

1 Chapter 22

2 Your Action Plan — The 30-Day Challenge

DISCLAIMER: This chapter is for educational and informational purposes only. It is not medical advice. The 30-day challenge described here is a framework for action, not a guaranteed protocol for curing cancer or eliminating parasites. Individual needs vary based on cancer type, stage, treatment status, organ function, and overall health. Some actions in this challenge may require medical supervision. Before starting any new testing, supplements, dietary changes, or medications, consult a qualified healthcare provider. This challenge is designed to be educational and empowering — not a substitute for professional medical care.

You've read 21 chapters. You've learned about parasites that cause cancer, drugs that might kill both, terrain theory, testing gaps, case studies, and communication strategies. You have more knowledge than 99% of cancer patients — and most oncologists — about the parasite-cancer connection.

Now what?

Knowledge without action is trivia. This chapter is your bridge from learning to doing. A 30-day roadmap. One action per day. Small steps. No overwhelm. Just forward motion.

2.1 Before You Start: The Commitment

The 30-day challenge is not about doing everything perfectly. It's about doing SOMETHING consistently. Pick the actions that fit your situation. Skip the ones that don't. Adapt as needed. The goal is momentum, not perfection.

If you're currently in active cancer treatment, some days will be harder than others. Fatigue, nausea, appointments, and emotional strain will interfere.

That's okay. Do what you can. Skip what you must. The challenge waits for you.

If you're post-treatment or in remission, this is your window for comprehensive terrain repair. Use it fully.

If you're a caregiver, do the challenge alongside your loved one. Your support makes the difference between "I tried" and "I did it."

2.2 Week 1: Foundation — Know Where You Stand

2.2.1 Day 1: Test Your pH

Buy pH test strips online or at a pharmacy. Test your first morning urine before eating or drinking. Record the number. Target: 6.5-7.5. If below 6.5, start the morning alkaline drink: warm water with lemon juice and a pinch of baking soda.

Why: pH is the single most accessible terrain marker. It tells you whether your internal environment favors parasites and cancer, or resists them.

2.2.2 Day 2: Assess Your Diet

For one day, write down everything you eat and drink. Mark each item: acid-forming (A) or alkaline-forming (AL). Count them. If acid-formers outnumber alkaline-formers by more than 2:1, you have work to do.

Why: Diet is the primary tool for terrain repair. You can't fix what you don't measure.

2.2.3 Day 3: Eliminate One Acid-Forming Food

Pick one: sugar, soda, processed snack, alcohol, or factory-farmed meat. Eliminate it for the rest of the challenge. Just one. Not all of them. One.

Why: Sustainable change happens one habit at a time. Cutting everything at once creates rebellion and failure.

2.2.4 Day 4: Add One Alkaline Food

Add one cup of leafy greens, one green smoothie, one serving of vegetables, or one alkaline fruit. Just one addition. Build from there.

Why: Addition is easier than subtraction. Crowd out the bad with the good.

2.2.5 Day 5: Hydration Audit

Measure your water intake for one day. Target: 2 liters of clean, filtered water. If you're below 1.5 liters, increase by one glass tomorrow.

Why: Hydration supports every detoxification pathway. Kidneys, colon, lymph, skin — all need water.

2.2.6 Day 6: Sleep Check

Track your sleep tonight. Time in bed, time asleep, awakenings, quality (1-10). Target: 7-9 hours of quality sleep. If you're below 6 hours or quality below 5, prioritize sleep hygiene tonight.

Why: Sleep is when the body repairs. Immune surveillance, DNA repair, detoxification — all peak during deep sleep.

2.2.7 Day 7: Stress Scan

Rate your stress level today (1-10). Identify the top three stressors. Write one thing you can do to reduce each — even slightly. Do one of them today.

Why: Chronic stress suppresses immunity and acidifies the body. Managing stress is not optional.

2.3 Week 2: Testing — Get the Data

2.3.1 Day 8: Research Parasite Testing in Your Area

Search for labs that offer comprehensive parasite testing. Options: - Your doctor's lab (if they'll order it) - Direct-to-consumer labs (if available in your region) - Functional medicine practitioners who offer testing - Major medical centers with parasitology departments

Why: You need data before you can act. Knowing what tests are available is the first step to getting them.

2.3.2 Day 9: Order or Request a Comprehensive Stool PCR Panel

This is the most important test in the challenge. A PCR stool panel detects: - Blastocystis - Cryptosporidium - Giardia - Dientamoeba fragilis - Entamoeba histolytica - Cyclospora - Helminth DNA (some panels) - Bacterial overgrowth markers

Why: PCR is 10-100x more sensitive than microscopy. The CDC confirms this. Don't settle for a basic O&P.

2.3.3 Day 10: Order or Request Parasite Serology

Blood tests for: - Echinococcus (hydatid disease) - Strongyloides stercoralis - Toxoplasma gondii - Schistosomiasis - Liver flukes (if risk factors present)

Why: Serology detects infections that stool tests miss — tissue parasites, dormant infections, and extrapulmonary disease.

2.3.4 Day 11: Get Vitamin D Tested

25-OH vitamin D. Target: 60-80 ng/mL. Most cancer patients are deficient. Most Americans are deficient in winter. Know your number.

Why: Vitamin D is essential for immune surveillance and cancer resistance. Deficiency is common and correctable.

2.3.5 Day 12: Get a Comprehensive Blood Panel

CBC, CMP, liver enzymes, inflammatory markers (CRP, ESR), ferritin, B12, folate, zinc, magnesium. These baseline markers track your terrain.

Why: You can't manage what you don't measure. Baseline labs guide your protocol and track progress.

2.3.6 Day 13: Document Your Symptoms

Write a symptom journal: energy, pain, digestion, sleep, mood, skin, urinary, bowel. Rate each (1-10). Date it. You'll compare this to Day 30.

Why: Subjective improvement matters. The journal turns vague feelings into trackable data.

2.3.7 Day 14: Read One Research Abstract

Search PubMed for one study mentioned in this book. Read the abstract. Not the whole paper — just the abstract. Understand what the researchers actually found.

Why: Self-education builds confidence. When you speak to doctors, speaking from direct knowledge changes the dynamic.

2.4 Week 3: Action — Start the Protocol

2.4.1 Day 15: Start Liver Support

Begin one liver-supportive practice: milk thistle (300-600 mg daily), dandelion tea, or a castor oil pack. Do it daily.

Why: Your liver processes everything — drugs, toxins, dead parasites. Support it before you start killing parasites.

2.4.2 Day 16: Begin a Probiotic

Start a multi-strain probiotic (50+ billion CFU). Take it daily, away from antiparasitic drugs if you start them later.

Why: Parasites disrupt gut bacteria. Antiparasitics disrupt them further. Rebuilding the microbiome is essential.

2.4.3 Day 17: Add One Herbal Antiparasitic

Choose one: wormwood, black walnut hull, cloves, oregano oil, or papaya seeds. Start with the lowest recommended dose. Take with food.

Why: Herbs target parasite life stages that drugs miss — especially eggs and cysts. They also have fewer side effects than pharmaceuticals.

2.4.4 Day 18: Dry Brushing and Movement

Start dry brushing (5 minutes before showering) and add one form of daily movement: walking, stretching, yoga, or rebounding.

Why: Lymphatic drainage and circulation support detoxification. Movement is medicine.

2.4.5 Day 19: Binder Introduction

If you're taking antiparasitics or herbs, add a binder: activated charcoal (500 mg, away from meds) or bentonite clay. This captures die-off toxins.

Why: Die-off reactions are real and miserable. Binders make them manageable.

2.4.6 Day 20: Discuss Antiparasitic Drugs with Your Doctor

If you have test results, or if your doctor is open to discussion, raise the question of pharmaceutical antiparasitics. Use the script from Chapter 21. Bring your evidence.

Why: Pharmaceutical antiparasitics are the most potent tools for confirmed infections. They're worth discussing if testing is positive or symptoms are strong.

2.4.7 Day 21: Deep Breathing Practice

Start a daily breathing practice: 5 minutes of slow, deep diaphragmatic breathing. Inhale for 4 counts, hold for 4, exhale for 6.

Why: Breathing alkalinizes the blood, reduces cortisol, improves oxygenation, and calms the nervous system. It's free and always available.

2.5 Week 4: Integration — Make It Stick

2.5.1 Day 22: Review Your pH Trend

Test your morning urine pH again. Compare to Day 1. Has it shifted? Even a 0.2-0.3 improvement is progress.

Why: pH changes slowly. Tracking the trend keeps you motivated when day-to-day variation is confusing.

2.5.2 Day 23: Evaluate Your Diet Shift

Look at your food log from Day 2. Compare to what you're eating now. Have you maintained the elimination and addition? Have alkaline foods increased?

Why: Diet is the foundation. Most people relapse here. The 3-week mark is when habits start to solidify.

2.5.3 Day 24: Check Test Results

If your parasite tests have returned, review them. What was found? What wasn't? What's the next step based on results?

Why: Data without action is useless. Results guide the next phase of your protocol.

2.5.4 Day 25: Add One Supplement Based on Deficiency

If your blood work showed low vitamin D, start D3. Low zinc, start zinc. Low magnesium, start magnesium. Targeted supplementation beats shotgun approaches.

Why: Nutrient repletion restores immune function and cellular repair. But only if you're actually deficient.

2.5.5 Day 26: Schedule Follow-Up Appointments

Book your follow-up with your oncologist, integrative practitioner, or infectious disease specialist. Bring your test results, symptom journal, and pH log.

Why: Follow-through separates people who gather information from people who use it.

2.5.6 Day 27: Share What You've Learned

Tell one person — family member, friend, or online community member — about what you've learned. Not to preach. Just to share.

Why: Teaching reinforces learning. And the person you tell might need this information someday.

2.5.7 Day 28: Review Your Symptom Journal

Compare your Day 13 symptom journal to today. What's improved? What's the same? What's worse? Write it down.

Why: 30 days is long enough to see changes — or to know that the current approach needs adjustment.

2.5.8 Day 29: Plan Your Maintenance Protocol

What will you continue after Day 30? The diet? The supplements? The testing schedule? The pH monitoring? Write your maintenance plan.

Why: The challenge ends. The work doesn't. Maintenance prevents backsliding.

2.5.9 Day 30: Celebrate and Commit

You've completed the 30-day challenge. Whether you did 10 actions or all 30, you've moved forward. Acknowledge the effort. Thank yourself for prioritizing your health. And commit to continuing.

Why: Momentum is everything. Day 30 is not the end. It's the beginning of a new baseline.

2.6 The Daily Non-Negotiables (Do These Every Day, Regardless of Everything Else)

1. **Hydration:** 2 liters clean water
2. **pH drink:** Morning lemon water or alkaline drink

3. **Movement:** Minimum 20 minutes walking or equivalent
4. **Sleep:** In bed with lights out at a consistent time
5. **One alkaline food:** Leafy greens, vegetables, or alkaline fruit
6. **One act of stress reduction:** Breathing, meditation, nature, music, connection

These six things take minimal time and cost minimal money. They form the foundation that everything else builds on.

2.7 The Weekly Checklist

Every Sunday, review: - [ ] pH tested 7 times this week - [ ] Diet log completed for at least 3 days - [ ] Supplements taken as scheduled - [ ] Movement completed 5+ days - [ ] Sleep quality rated nightly - [ ] Symptoms journaled - [ ] One educational action completed (reading, video, conversation) - [ ] Practitioners contacted if needed

The checklist keeps you honest. It's your weekly audit.

2.8 What If You're Overwhelmed?

The 30-day challenge assumes energy, time, and capacity that many cancer patients don't have. If you're overwhelmed:

Do the Week 1 actions only. pH, diet, hydration, sleep, stress. That's it. These five things — done consistently — change your terrain more than any drug.

Add one action per week, not per day. Days 8-30 can be spread over months. The timeline doesn't matter. The direction matters.

Delegate. Ask your caregiver to research testing options. Ask your partner to prepare alkaline meals. Ask a friend to remind you about supplements. You don't have to do everything yourself.

Lower the bar. If you can't do 20 minutes of movement, do 5 minutes. If you can't eliminate sugar completely, cut it in half. If you can't test pH daily, test it once a week. Something is always better than nothing.

2.9 What You Can Do Today

1. Print this chapter.

Put it on your refrigerator. Put it in your medical binder. Make it visible. The 30-day challenge doesn't work if it's buried in a PDF on your computer.

2. Circle the three actions that feel most doable right now.

Not the most important. The most doable. The ones you'll actually do. Start there.

3. Set one alarm on your phone.

For pH testing. For supplements. For movement. For bedtime. One alarm. One reminder. One habit at a time.

4. Text one person: "I'm starting a 30-day health challenge. Will you check in with me weekly?"

Accountability works. Social support works. Use them.

5. Write this sentence in your journal: "I am taking the second look."

It's not just a book title. It's a decision. A commitment. A declaration that you're not settling for the standard playbook when your life is on the line.

Sources & Evidence Tiers for This Chapter:

Claim	Evidence	Tier
pH testing is an accessible terrain marker	Biological plausibility	**Plausible**
Dietary change affects inflammation and immunity	Nutritional science	**Established**
Hydration supports detoxification	Physiology	**Established**

Claim	Evidence	Tier
Sleep quality affects immune function	Sleep medicine	**Established**
Stress management reduces cortisol and inflammation	Psychoneuroimmunology	**Established**
Probiotics support gut health after antiparasitic treatment	Meta-analyses	**Established**
This specific 30-day protocol has not been validated in RCTs	Absence of trials	**Not Proven**

Full references with URLs and DOIs are available in Appendix G.

Bonus Chapter: Parasites and Diabetes — What the Evidence Actually Shows

Chapter X — Bonus Material

What This Chapter Covers

The relationship between parasitic infections and diabetes is one of the most misunderstood topics in both alternative health circles and conventional medicine. Some claim parasites *cause* diabetes. Others dismiss any connection entirely. The truth, backed by peer-reviewed research, is more nuanced — and more interesting — than either extreme. This chapter presents what is actually proven, what is merely possible, and what remains unproven, using only verifiable studies from PubMed, Nature, and other indexed sources.

The Core Finding: Diabetic Patients Have Higher Rates of Parasites

The strongest, most consistently replicated finding across multiple meta-analyses is this: **people with diabetes have a higher prevalence of intestinal parasitic infections than people without diabetes.**

The 2024 Meta-Analysis: Taghipour et al.

A systematic review and meta-analysis published in *International Health* (2024) analyzed 22 studies — thirteen case-control and nine cross-sectional — to evaluate the pooled prevalence and odds ratio of intestinal parasitic infections (IPIs) in diabetic patients. The results were significant:

- **Overall pooled prevalence of IPIs in diabetic patients: 24.4%** (95% CI 18.8%–31%)
- **Case-control comparison:** 25.7% in diabetic patients vs. 15.5% in controls
- **Odds ratio:** OR 1.80 (95% CI 1.08–2.97) — diabetic patients had nearly double the odds of carrying intestinal parasites

This is not fringe science. This is a PRISMA-protocol systematic review published by Oxford University Press on behalf of the Royal Society of Tropical Medicine and Hygiene.

What This Proves — And What It Does Not

Proven: Diabetic patients, particularly in endemic regions, carry intestinal parasites at measurably higher rates than non-diabetic controls.

Not proven: That the parasites *caused* the diabetes. The direction of causality is unresolved. Diabetes itself impairs immune function, alters gut motility, changes microbiome composition, and increases susceptibility to infection. A diabetic patient may be *more likely to acquire* parasites, not the other way around.

> **Learn from This Mistake:** The correlation-versus-causation trap. Just because two things occur together does not mean one caused the other. High parasite rates in diabetics could mean parasites cause diabetes, diabetes causes vulnerability to parasites, or both are caused by a third factor (poverty, poor sanitation, immune dysfunction). Be precise in your claims.

Specific Parasites: The Evidence Breakdown

Cryptosporidium — The Strongest Association

The 2024 Taghipour meta-analysis found **Cryptosporidium** to be significantly more common in diabetic patients, with an odds ratio of **3.30** (95% CI 1.86–5.86). This is one of the strongest single-parasite associations in the literature.

Cryptosporidium causes severe, persistent diarrhea, dehydration, malabsorption, and weight loss. In a diabetic patient, chronic diarrhea and dehydration can destabilize blood glucose control, trigger diabetic ketoacidosis in Type 1 patients, and worsen overall metabolic stability.

Clinical relevance: High. **Causation proof:** None. The association is robust; causation is unproven.

Blastocystis — Controversial but Frequent

The same meta-analysis found **Blastocystis** significantly more common in diabetic patients, OR **1.57** (95% CI 1.11–2.22).

Blastocystis is controversial because many carriers are asymptomatic. However, it is one of the most frequently studied organisms in gut inflammation, microbiome disruption, and metabolic disease research. Some studies link it to irritable bowel syndrome; others find no pathology at all.

Evidence strength: Weak to moderate association. Clinical significance remains debated.

Hookworm — Mixed Evidence

The 2024 meta-analysis found hookworm associated with diabetes at OR **6.09** (95% CI 1.11–33.41). The extremely wide confidence interval signals high uncertainty — the true effect could be minimal or very large.

However, hookworm presents a fascinating paradox. While infection-prevalence studies show association, **controlled therapeutic trials suggest hookworm may actually improve**

insulin resistance.

The Paradox: Some Parasites May Protect Against Diabetes

This is the part that surprises most people. A substantial body of research — including randomized controlled trials — suggests that certain helminth (worm) infections may *reduce* insulin resistance and protect against Type 2 diabetes through immune modulation.

The Indonesia SUGARSPIN Trial (2017)

The SUGARSPIN trial was a household-cluster-randomized, double-blind, placebo-controlled clinical trial conducted on Flores Island, Indonesia — an area endemic for soil-transmitted helminths. 1,669 subjects were examined across albendazole and placebo arms.

Key findings: - Albendazole (deworming) reduced helminth prevalence, total IgE, and eosinophil count as expected - At the **community level**, deworming had no effect on insulin resistance - Among **helminth-infected subjects specifically**, deworming **significantly increased insulin resistance** (treatment effect 0.031, 95% CI 0.004–0.059, P = 0.04) - The interaction P-value was 0.01 — the effect was specific to infected individuals

What this means: Removing helminth infections from already-infected people made their metabolic health *worse*. The parasites appeared to be providing a protective metabolic effect.

A follow-up analysis of the same trial population (published in *Nutrition & Diabetes*, 2017) found that deworming in infected subjects increased the leptin-to-adiponectin ratio — a marker associated with worse metabolic health — and this partially mediated the insulin resistance increase.

The Australian Controlled Hookworm Trial (2023)

A study published in *Nature Communications* examined **experimental hookworm infection** in people at risk of Type 2 diabetes. Participants were deliberately infected with low-dose hookworm larvae and monitored over two years.

Results: The hookworm group showed **improvements in fasting blood glucose and insulin resistance after one year**, with a reduction in body weight observed after two years. Adverse events were more frequent in the hookworm group, but completion rates were similar.

This is one of the few human studies of deliberate helminth infection for metabolic disease — and the results support the protective hypothesis.

The Chinese Schistosoma Study (2013)

A large cross-sectional study published in the *Journal of Clinical Endocrinology & Metabolism* examined 9,539 participants aged 40+ in rural China, including 463 with previous schistosome infection (PSI).

Striking results: - Diabetes prevalence: **14.9%** in PSI group vs. **25.4%** in uninfected controls (P < 0.0001) - Metabolic syndrome prevalence: **14.0%** in PSI group vs. **35.0%** in controls (P < 0.0001) - Adjusted odds ratio for diabetes with PSI: **0.51** (95% CI 0.34–0.77) — a **49% reduction in risk** - PSI participants also had significantly lower fasting glucose, postprandial glucose, HbA1c, and HOMA-IR

This protective association persisted after adjustment for age, sex, BMI, and diet. The authors concluded: "If confirmed, the protecting effect of helminth infection could be reconsidered in terms of therapeutic strategies."

Mouse Studies and Mechanism

Animal studies show helminth infection or helminth-derived products can: - Improve insulin sensitivity - Reduce systemic inflammation - Alter gut microbiota toward beneficial profiles - Increase regulatory immune responses (Tregs) - Improve glucose metabolism

A 2021 review assessed fourteen studies: nine reported protective effects of helminth infection on diabetes-related parameters, three reported positive associations with T2D diagnosis, and two reported no association.

Evidence strength for protection: Moderate. The human RCT data (SUGARSPIN, hookworm trial) and large epidemiological studies (Chinese schistosoma) are compelling. However, this is **not a recommendation to infect yourself with parasites.**

Toxoplasma gondii — The Protozoan Suspect

Toxoplasma gondii is one of the most studied parasites in diabetes research because it infects pancreatic tissue in animal models and has been epidemiologically linked to both Type 1 and Type 2 diabetes.

Type 1 Diabetes

A 2023 systematic review and meta-analysis examined the association between *T. gondii* and Type 1 diabetes mellitus. The authors noted the subject remains controversial and limited by small study numbers.

An experimental study (2018) found that chronically *T. gondii*-infected animals showed **reduced insulin expression in pancreatic islets and increased serum glucose** — though full diabetes did not develop during the study period. This suggests a biological mechanism is plausible: the parasite may damage insulin-producing cells.

Type 2 Diabetes

A 2025 meta-analysis (Catchpole et al., *Folia Parasitologica*) included **25 studies** with 4,639 Type 2 diabetes patients and 3,492 controls. The biological theory is that *T. gondii* may affect pancreatic tissue, immune signaling, or systemic inflammation. If the parasite damages pancreatic cells, it could theoretically impair insulin secretion.

Evidence strength: Mixed association. *T. gondii* is a plausible risk factor, but the epidemiological data is inconsistent and no causal pathway has been definitively established in humans.

Strongyloides stercoralis — A Special Case

Strongyloides presents a complex picture. A 2024 meta-analysis found a significant association between *Strongyloides stercoralis* infection and diabetes — but in the **protective direction**. Infected individuals were **less likely** to develop diabetes, potentially supporting the "hygiene hypothesis."

However, there is a critical clinical point for diabetic patients: **Strongyloides hyperinfection syndrome.** In diabetic patients, or anyone receiving steroids, chemotherapy, or immune-suppressing medications, latent Strongyloides can transform into a life-threatening hyperinfection. This is not a theoretical risk — it is a well-documented, often fatal complication.

Even if Strongyloides may not cause diabetes, it demands attention in any immunocompromised or diabetic patient with exposure history.

The Rare Exception: Pancreatic Parasites

There are documented case reports where parasites in or near the pancreas have caused pancreatitis and **secondary diabetes** — diabetes resulting from pancreatic damage rather than autoimmune or insulin resistance mechanisms.

A 2019 case report in the *Indian Journal of Medical Specialities*, titled "Worm Causing Diabetes," described a patient with a **pancreatic hydatid cyst** (caused by *Echinococcus* tapeworm larvae) who developed pancreatitis and subsequent diabetes. Surgical removal of the cyst addressed both conditions.

This is important but rare. It is case-report evidence, not proof that parasites commonly cause diabetes. Hydatid cysts in the pancreas are uncommon, and secondary diabetes from parasitic pancreatitis is an outlier, not a pattern.

Evidence Summary Table

Parasite / Group	Diabetes Connection	Evidence Type	Direction	Strength
Intestinal parasites overall	Higher prevalence in diabetic patients	Systematic reviews / meta-analyses	Diabetes associated with more parasites	**Moderate**
Cryptosporidium	More common in diabetics; worsens diarrhea/dehydration	Meta-analysis	Possible worsening / infection risk	**Moderate**
Blastocystis	More common in diabetic patients	Meta-analysis	Association	**Weak–Moderate**
Hookworm	Associated in prevalence studies; improved insulin resistance in RCTs	Meta-analysis / human trial	Mixed; may protect insulin sensitivity	**Mixed**
Toxoplasma gondii	Studied in T1D and T2D; possible pancreatic effect	Meta-analyses / animal studies	Possible risk factor	**Mixed**
Strongyloides stercoralis	Clinically important in diabetics; may be inversely associated	Human studies / meta-analysis	Mixed / possibly protective	**Mixed**
Schistosoma	Previous infection associated with dramatically lower diabetes rates	Large cross-sectional study (n=9,539)	Often protective	**Moderate**
Echinococcus / pancreatic hydatid cyst	Rare pancreatitis → secondary diabetes	Case reports only	Rare possible cause	**Weak / case-only**

What Is Proven vs. What Is Not

Strongly Supported by Evidence

- People with diabetes have higher prevalence of intestinal parasitic infections in multiple meta-analyses (pooled prevalence ~24–26%).
- Diabetes itself increases vulnerability to infections through immune dysfunction, gut changes, and metabolic stress.
- Some parasites (Cryptosporidium) can worsen diarrhea, dehydration, and blood sugar instability in diabetic patients.
- Certain helminths — particularly hookworm and schistosome — are associated with **better** metabolic outcomes and lower diabetes risk in controlled studies.

- *Toxoplasma gondii* has plausible biological mechanisms for affecting pancreatic function, but human causation is unproven.

Possible But Not Proven

- *T. gondii* may contribute to pancreatic islet dysfunction and diabetes risk.
- Some protozoa may worsen metabolic inflammation.
- Parasite treatment may improve health outcomes in infected diabetic patients (reasonable clinical practice, but not universally proven).
- Rare pancreatic parasites may damage the pancreas enough to cause secondary diabetes.

Not Proven — And Likely False

- "All diabetes is caused by parasites."
- "All diabetics have pancreatic flukes."
- "Killing parasites cures diabetes."
- "Parasites are the main cause of Type 2 diabetes."
- "Helminth therapy should be standard diabetes treatment." (Promising research; not clinical standard.)

Practical Implications for Patients and Clinicians

Should Diabetic Patients Be Screened for Parasites?

Based on the evidence, **yes — in specific circumstances:**

- Persistent gastrointestinal symptoms (diarrhea, bloating, malabsorption)
- Unexplained eosinophilia on blood work
- Travel or residence in endemic regions
- Immune suppression or steroid use
- Unexplained weight loss or anemia
- Poor glycemic control despite standard management

The 2024 meta-analysis authors explicitly recommend: "proper health education program and preventing measures for the acquisition of IPIs in patients with diabetes."

Should Patients Deliberately Infect Themselves With Helminths?

No. The protective helminth studies are research data, not clinical recommendations. Experimental helminth infection carries risks: anemia, gastrointestinal symptoms, allergic responses, and unknown long-term effects. The Australian hookworm trial reported more adverse events in the hookworm group. Do not attempt this outside a controlled clinical trial.

The Bottom Line

The relationship between parasites and diabetes is **bidirectional and complex:**

1. Diabetes increases susceptibility to intestinal parasites.
2. Some parasites (Cryptosporidium) worsen diabetic symptoms and stability.
3. Some parasites (*T. gondii*) are plausible but unproven contributors to diabetes risk.
4. Some helminths appear to **protect** against Type 2 diabetes through immune modulation.
5. Rare pancreatic parasites can cause secondary diabetes via pancreatitis.

There is no single narrative. The evidence does not support "parasites cause diabetes" as a universal claim. It supports a nuanced, context-dependent relationship that varies by parasite species, host immune status, and geographic setting.

> **Learn from This Mistake:** A patient in an online forum read that "all diabetes is caused by parasites" and spent thousands on unproven parasite cleanses, delaying actual medical care. By the time they saw an endocrinologist, their HbA1c was 14.2%. Parasite screening has a place in comprehensive diabetes care — but it is not a replacement for evidence-based diabetes management.

Chapter Summary

- **Proven:** Diabetic patients have higher rates of intestinal parasites (~24% pooled prevalence).
- **Proven:** Some helminths may protect against Type 2 diabetes via immune modulation (SUGARSPIN trial, Chinese schistosoma study, Australian hookworm trial).
- **Possible:** *Toxoplasma gondii* may be a risk factor for diabetes through pancreatic effects.
- **Not proven:** Parasites are the primary cause of diabetes, or deworming cures diabetes.
- **Actionable:** Diabetic patients with GI symptoms, travel history, or immune suppression should consider parasite screening as part of comprehensive care.

Sources and References

The following sources were used in the preparation of this chapter and are provided for independent verification:

1. **Taghipour A, et al.** "Prevalence of intestinal parasitic infections in patients with diabetes: a systematic review and meta-analysis." *International Health.* 2024;16(1):23–33. PMID: 37052134.
https://pubmed.ncbi.nlm.nih.gov/37052134/

2. **Anywar DA, et al.** "Prevalence and factors associated with Intestinal parasitosis among adults with diabetes mellitus attending a tertiary care facility in Northern Uganda." *PLoS Neglected Tropical Diseases.* 2025. PMCID: PMC12742753. https://pmc.ncbi.nlm.nih.gov/articles/PMC12742753/

3. **Catchpole A, et al.** "Association between type-2 diabetes and Toxoplasma gondii seropositivity: a systematic review and meta-analysis." *Folia Parasitologica.* 2025;72:2025.024. PMID: 40910161.
https://pubmed.ncbi.nlm.nih.gov/40910161/

4. **Pierce DR, et al.** "Effect of experimental hookworm infection on insulin resistance in people at risk of type 2 diabetes." *Nature Communications.* 2023;14:40263.
https://www.nature.com/articles/s41467-023-40263-4

5. **Tiongco RE, et al.** "Association of Strongyloides stercoralis infection with the development of diabetes mellitus: a meta-analysis." *PubMed.* 2024. PMID: 39703057.
https://pubmed.ncbi.nlm.nih.gov/39703057/

6. **Singh A.** "Worm Causing Diabetes." *Indian Journal of Medical Specialities.* 2019;10(4).
https://journals.lww.com/imsp/fulltext/2019/10020/worm_causing_diabetes.12.aspx

7. **Tahapary DL, et al.** "Effect of Anthelmintic Treatment on Insulin Resistance: A Cluster-Randomized, Placebo-Controlled Trial in Indonesia." *Clinical Infectious Diseases.* 2017;65(5):764–771. PMID: 28472383.
https://pubmed.ncbi.nlm.nih.gov/28472383/

8. **Tahapary DL, et al.** "Effect of anthelmintic treatment on leptin, adiponectin and leptin to adiponectin ratio: a randomized-controlled trial." *Nutrition & Diabetes.* 2017;7:e289.
https://pmc.ncbi.nlm.nih.gov/articles/PMC5678209/

9. **Chen Y, et al.** "Association of previous schistosome infection with diabetes and metabolic syndrome: a cross-sectional study in rural China." *Journal of Clinical Endocrinology & Metabolism.* 2013;98(2):E283–E287. PMID: 23275524.
https://pubmed.ncbi.nlm.nih.gov/23275524/

10. **Shen S-W, et al.** "The potential long-term effect of previous schistosome infection reduces the risk of metabolic syndrome among Chinese men." *Parasite Immunology.* 2015;37(7):333–339. PMID: 25809087.
https://pubmed.ncbi.nlm.nih.gov/25809087/

11. **Zhu Y, et al.** "Clinical challenges and technological breakthroughs in helminthic therapy for diabetes." *Frontiers in Immunology.* 2025;16:1642707.
https://www.frontiersin.org/journals/immunology/articles/10.3389/fimmu.2025.1642707/full

---

This chapter was compiled from peer-reviewed, indexed medical literature. All URLs were verified at the time of writing. Readers are encouraged to review the original sources for full methodology, statistical detail, and author conclusions.

Appendix A: The IARC Parasite-Carcinogen Classifications

A Quick Reference

The **International Agency for Research on Cancer (IARC)** classifies agents into groups based on the strength of evidence that they cause cancer in humans. This appendix lists the parasite-related classifications.

IARC Group 1: Carcinogenic to Humans — PROVEN

These parasites have sufficient evidence of carcinogenicity in humans.

Parasite	Cancer Caused	Primary Location	Evidence Source
Schistosoma haematobium	Bladder squamous cell carcinoma	Bladder, ureters	IARC Monographs Vol. 61 (1994)
Opisthorchis viverrini	Cholangiocarcinoma (bile duct cancer)	Bile ducts, liver	IARC Monographs Vol. 61 (1994)
Clonorchis sinensis	Cholangiocarcinoma	Bile ducts, liver	IARC Monographs Vol. 100B (2012)

What Group 1 means: The evidence is as strong as it gets. Same category as asbestos, tobacco smoke, and plutonium. These parasites definitively cause cancer in humans.

IARC Group 2A: Probably Carcinogenic to Humans

Limited evidence in humans, but sufficient evidence in animals or strong mechanistic data.

Parasite	Cancer Association	Primary Location	Notes
Plasmodium falciparum	Burkitt lymphoma (with EBV co-infection)	Lymphatic system	Malaria + EBV synergy; IARC Group 2A
Clonorchis sinensis	Cholangiocarcinoma	Liver/bile ducts	Some classifications list as Group 2A; upgraded to Group 1 in Vol. 100B

What Group 2A means: Probably causes cancer in humans. The evidence is strong but not as extensive as Group 1.

IARC Group 2B: Possibly Carcinogenic to Humans

Limited evidence in humans and less than sufficient evidence in animals.

Parasite	Cancer Association	Primary Location	Notes
Schistosoma japonicum	Colorectal cancer	Colon, rectum	Limited evidence; some studies suggest association

Parasite	Cancer Association	Primary Location	Notes
Schistosoma mansoni	Colorectal cancer (possible)	Colon, rectum	Less studied than S. japonicum

What Group 2B means: Possibly carcinogenic. The evidence exists but is limited or inconsistent.

IARC Group 3: Not Classifiable

Inadequate evidence in humans and animals.

Parasite	Cancer Association	Notes
Opisthorchis felineus	Not classifiable	Related to O. viverrini but insufficient human data
Other trematodes	Not classifiable	Many species lack sufficient study

What Group 3 means: Not enough data to classify. This does NOT mean "safe" — it means "we don't know yet."

Key Points to Remember

1. **Only three parasites are PROVEN (Group 1) carcinogens:** S. haematobium, O. viverrini, and C. sinensis. These are liver flukes and blood flukes.
2. **Group 1 = undeniable.** When someone says "parasites don't cause cancer," the WHO disagrees. In the same way it disagrees about smoking.

3. **Many parasites are NOT classified** simply because nobody has studied them for carcinogenicity. IARC only evaluates agents with sufficient research. The absence of classification does not mean safety.
4. **Malaria + EBV = lymphoma.** The Plasmodium falciparum-Burkitt lymphoma link (Group 2A) is one of the best-studied parasite-cancer interactions, demonstrating how parasites can create the conditions for cancer without directly causing it.

How IARC Classification Works

Group	Meaning	Examples
Group 1	Carcinogenic to humans	Tobacco, asbestos, S. haematobium, O. viverrini, C. sinensis, HPV, H. pylori
Group 2A	Probably carcinogenic	Red meat, shift work, P. falciparum (with EBV)
Group 2B	Possibly carcinogenic	Coffee, pickled vegetables, S. japonicum
Group 3	Not classifiable	Tea, fluorescent lighting, O. felineus
Group 4	Probably NOT carcinogenic	Caprolactam (only one example)

Source: IARC Monographs Programme, World Health Organization. https://monographs.iarc.who.int/

The Parasite-Cancer Connection Appendix A - IARC Parasite-Carcinogen Classifications

Appendix B: Common Parasites and Their Cancer Associations

Quick Reference Table

Parasite	Type	Body Part Affected	Cancer Link	Evidence Level	Key Study / Source
Schistosoma haematobium	Blood fluke (trematode)	Bladder, ureters, genitals	Bladder squamous cell carcinoma	**PROVEN (IARC Group 1)**	IARC Monographs Vol. 61 (1994)
Opisthorchis viverrini	Liver fluke (trematode)	Bile ducts, liver	Cholangiocarcinoma	**PROVEN (IARC Group 1)**	IARC Monographs Vol. 61 (1994); Sripa et al., PLoS Med 2007
Clonorchis sinensis	Liver fluke (trematode)	Bile ducts, liver	Cholangiocarcinoma	**PROVEN (IARC Group 1)**	IARC Monographs Vol. 100B (2012)
Schistosoma japonicum	Blood fluke (trematode)	Colon, rectum, liver	Colorectal cancer (possible)	Possible (IARC Group 2B)	Limited epidemiological data
Plasmodium falciparum	Protozoa	Blood, liver (acute), lymphatic system (chronic)	Burkitt lymphoma (with EBV)	Probable (IARC Group 2A)	Malaria-lymphoma epidemiology in Africa
Toxoplasma gondii	Protozoa	Brain, muscle, eyes	Glioma (brain cancer) - modest association	Emerging	Su et al. meta-analysis, 2021
Trichomonas vaginalis	Protozoa	Urogenital tract	Prostate cancer - aggressive forms	Moderate / Conflicting	Hodge et al. meta-analysis, 2019; mixed results
Blastocystis	Protozoa	Intestine	Colorectal cancer associations	Emerging	Multiple recent studies

Parasite	Type	Body Part Affected	Cancer Link	Evidence Level	Key Study / Source
Echinococcus granulosus / multilocularis	Tapeworm (cestode)	Liver, lung, brain, bone, kidney	Tumor mimic - misdiagnosed as cancer	Established (radiology)	"Great Neoplasms Mimicker" - Craig et al.
Hymenolepis nana	Tapeworm (cestode)	Intestine	Direct malignant transformation (rare)	Verified case report	NEJM 2015 - Muehlenbachs et al.
Strongyloides stercoralis	Roundworm (nematode)	Intestine, lungs, skin	Hyperinfection syndrome in cancer patients (fatal)	Established	CDC guidance; clinical parasitology
Giardia lamblia	Protozoa	Small intestine	Chronic malabsorption; links to lymphoproliferative disorders (rare)	Weak / Rare	Case reports only
Cryptosporidium	Protozoa	Intestine	Chronic infection in immunocompromised; cholangiocarcinoma in AIDS patients	Rare / Immunocompromised	Case reports in HIV/AIDS populations
Fasciola hepatica	Liver fluke (trematode)	Bile ducts, liver	Bile duct hyperplasia; possible cholangiocarcinoma link	Emerging / Animal data	Veterinary studies; limited human data

Notes on Evidence Levels

PROVEN (IARC Group 1): Sufficient evidence in humans. No reasonable doubt.

Probable (IARC Group 2A): Strong evidence but not yet definitive.

Possible (IARC Group 2B): Limited or inconsistent evidence.

Emerging: New research, promising but preliminary.

Moderate / Conflicting: Some studies find associations, others do not.

Established (non-carcinogenic): Echinococcus does not cause cancer but is a master tumor mimic - critical for differential diagnosis.

High-Risk Parasites for Cancer Patients

If you have cancer or are immunocompromised, these parasites pose the greatest direct threat:

1. **Strongyloides stercoralis** - Chemotherapy and steroids can trigger fatal hyperinfection.
2. **Cryptosporidium** - Immunocompromised patients develop chronic, debilitating infection.
3. **Toxoplasma gondii** - Already present in 30-50% of population; reactivation risk during immunosuppression.
4. **Echinococcus** - If you have a "tumor" in liver, lung, or bone, demand ruling out hydatid cyst before biopsy.

Appendix C: Antiparasitic Dosage Quick Reference

For Discussion with Your Doctor

IMPORTANT: The dosages below are standard **antiparasitic doses** used for treating worm and protozoal infections. Using these drugs for **cancer** is off-label, experimental, and not FDA-approved. Always consult a qualified healthcare provider before taking any medication.

Prescription Antiparasitics

Ivermectin

Indication	Dose	Duration	Notes
Strongyloidiasis	200 mcg/kg once daily	1-2 days	Repeat in 2 weeks if needed
Onchocerciasis	150 mcg/kg once	Single dose	Co-administer with doxycycline for Wolbachia
Scabies	200 mcg/kg once	Repeat in 7-14 days	Often combined with permethrin cream
General parasite cleanse (off-label)	200 mcg/kg weekly	4-8 weeks	**Experimental for cancer — discuss with doctor**

Safety profile: Exceptionally safe. Billions of doses administered. Caution in patients with meningitis or heavy Loa loa co-infection (rare encephalopathy risk).

Albendazole

Indication	Dose	Duration	Notes
Echinococcosis (hydatid disease)	400 mg twice daily	28 days + surgical intervention	Often combined with praziquantel
Neurocysticercosis	400 mg twice daily	8-30 days	Requires steroid cover to manage inflammation
Hookworm, roundworm	400 mg once	Single dose	May repeat in 2 weeks
General antiparasitic	400 mg daily	3-5 days	With fatty meal for absorption

Safety profile: Generally well-tolerated. Monitor liver enzymes. Teratogenic — avoid in pregnancy.

Mebendazole

Indication	Dose	Duration	Notes
Pinworm	100 mg once	Single dose; repeat in 2 weeks	Treat entire household
Roundworm, hookworm, whipworm	100 mg twice daily	3 days	Chewable tablet
General antiparasitic	100-200 mg twice daily	3-5 days	Available over-the-counter in some countries

Safety profile: Very safe. Minimal side effects. First-line for pinworm especially in children.

Praziquantel

Indication	Dose	Duration	Notes
Schistosomiasis	40 mg/kg (divided into 2 doses)	Single day	Take with food and fluids
Liver flukes (Opisthorchis, Clonorchis)	25 mg/kg three times daily	1-2 days	May cause abdominal discomfort
Tapeworms (cestodes)	5-10 mg/kg once	Single dose	Cysticercosis requires specialist management

Safety profile: Well-tolerated. Common side effect: abdominal cramping as parasites die. Contraindicated in ocular cysticercosis (inflammation can blind).

Nitazoxanide

Indication	Dose	Duration	Notes
Cryptosporidiosis	500 mg twice daily	3 days	First-line for immunocompetent patients
Giardiasis	500 mg twice daily	3 days	Alternative to metronidazole
General protozoal infections	500 mg twice daily	3-7 days	Broad-spectrum antiprotozoal

Safety profile: Generally well-tolerated. Available in liquid form for children.

Veterinary Antiparasitics (Not for Human Use Without Medical Supervision)

Fenbendazole

Animal Use	Human Use Status
Dogs: 50 mg/kg daily for 3 days Off-label cancer discussion	**NOT FDA-approved for humans** Doses discussed in online communities range from 222 mg/day ("Joe Tippens protocol") to higher amounts — **NO established human safety data**

CRITICAL WARNING: Fenbendazole is a veterinary drug. Human pharmacokinetics, safety, and efficacy are unknown. Do not self-administer. If interested, discuss with an oncologist familiar with off-label antiparasitic research.

Natural / Herbal Antiparasitics

These are **supplements**, not drugs. Quality varies dramatically by brand. Use reputable sources.

Supplement	Typical Dose	Notes
Wormwood (Artemisia absinthium)	300-500 mg extract, 1-3x daily	Traditional antiparasitic; contains thujone — avoid high doses long-term
Black walnut hull	500-1000 mg, 1-3x daily	Traditionally used for intestinal worms
Cloves (Syzygium aromaticum)	500 mg, 1-3x daily	Target parasite eggs; often used with wormwood/black walnut

Supplement	Typical Dose	Notes
Pumpkin seeds	1-2 cups raw seeds daily	Traditional remedy for tapeworms; limited modern evidence
Diatomaceous earth (food grade)	1 teaspoon in water daily	Mechanical parasite removal; drink plenty of water
Papaya seeds	1 tablespoon daily	Traditional use; some studies show antiparasitic activity
Garlic	2-4 cloves raw daily	General antimicrobial; traditional antiparasitic
Oregano oil	200-500 mg daily	Broad antimicrobial; capsules preferred over liquid (burns)

Key Safety Notes

1. **Pregnancy:** Most antiparasitics are contraindicated. Pyrantel pamoate is often considered safest in pregnancy, but only under medical supervision.
2. **Liver disease:** Albendazole and mebendazole require liver monitoring. Use caution with existing liver conditions.
3. **Immunocompromised:** Strongyloides hyperinfection risk is REAL. Test and treat BEFORE starting chemotherapy or steroids.

4. **Drug interactions:** Ivermectin is a CYP3A4 substrate. Check interactions with other medications.
5. **Children:** Dosing is weight-based for children. Do not use adult doses.
6. **Self-treatment risks:** Misdiagnosis, incorrect drug choice, inadequate dosing, and failure to treat household contacts can lead to reinfection.

Questions to Ask Your Doctor

- "Given my diagnosis, should I be tested for parasites before starting treatment?"
- "Which antiparasitic is safest with my current medications?"
- "If we find parasites, should we treat them before, during, or after cancer treatment?"
- "Are there drug interaction concerns with my chemotherapy regimen?"
- "Should my family members also be tested?"

The Parasite-Cancer Connection Appendix C — Antiparasitic Dosage Quick Reference

Appendix D: pH Food Chart — Acid vs. Alkaline

How to Use This Chart

This chart classifies foods by their **effect on body pH after digestion**, not by their taste. Lemons taste acidic but have an **alkaline-forming** effect in the body. Meat tastes savory but is **acid-forming**.

The goal: Shift your diet toward 70-80% alkaline-forming foods and 20-30% acid-forming foods. First morning urine pH target: 6.5-7.5.

Highly Alkaline-Forming Foods (Eat More)

Food Category	Examples
Leafy greens	Spinach, kale, Swiss chard, collards, romaine lettuce, arugula, dandelion greens
Cruciferous vegetables	Broccoli, cauliflower, Brussels sprouts, cabbage, bok choy
Other vegetables	Cucumber, celery, zucchini, bell peppers, asparagus, green beans, okra
Root vegetables	Beets (raw), carrots, sweet potatoes, yams, radishes
Alkalizing fruits	Lemons, limes, grapefruit, watermelon, cantaloupe, mango, papaya, avocado
Sprouts	Alfalfa, broccoli sprouts, mung bean sprouts, wheatgrass, barley grass
Alkaline water	pH 8-9 (with minerals); add lemon or a pinch of baking soda to filtered water
Green drinks	Chlorophyll, spirulina, chlorella, wheatgrass juice

Food Category	Examples
Herbs & spices	Ginger, turmeric, garlic, cilantro, parsley, basil, cayenne
Almonds & almond milk	Raw almonds; unsweetened almond milk
Cold-pressed oils	Olive oil, flaxseed oil, coconut oil (small amounts)

Moderately Alkaline-Forming Foods (Eat Regularly)

Food Category	Examples
Most fruits	Apples, pears, berries, peaches, plums, cherries, grapes, kiwi, bananas (ripe)
Most vegetables	Tomatoes, onions, mushrooms, eggplant, squash, artichokes, leeks
Legumes	Lentils, green peas, edamame (fresh soybeans)
Seeds	Pumpkin seeds, sunflower seeds, sesame seeds, flaxseeds, chia seeds
Herbal teas	Chamomile, peppermint, ginger, dandelion, rooibos
Fermented foods	Sauerkraut (unpasteurized), kimchi, miso (small amounts), coconut kefir

---

Neutral / Mildly Acidic Foods (Eat in Moderation)

Food Category	Examples
Most grains	Brown rice, quinoa, oats, millet, buckwheat, amaranth (whole, unprocessed)
Beans	Black beans, kidney beans, chickpeas, navy beans
Nuts (except almonds)	Walnuts, cashews, pistachios, pecans, macadamia
Most oils	Sesame oil, sunflower oil (avoid industrial seed oils)
Organic tofu & tempeh	Non-GMO, organic sources only
Natural sweeteners	Raw honey (small amounts), pure maple syrup, stevia, monk fruit

---

Highly Acid-Forming Foods (Reduce or Eliminate)

Food Category	Examples	Why It Matters
Processed meats	Bacon, sausage, hot dogs, deli meats, ham	Nitrates, high omega-6, inflammatory
Red meat	Beef, pork, lamb (especially grain-fed)	High arachidonic acid, acidifying
Conventional dairy	Milk, cheese, yogurt, ice cream (non-organic)	Acidifying; often contains hormones and antibiotics
Refined grains	White bread, white rice, pasta, pastries	Strip of alkalizing minerals; spike insulin
Sugar	White sugar, high-fructose corn syrup, candy, soda	Feeds parasites and cancer cells; highly acidifying
Artificial sweeteners	Aspartame, sucralose, saccharin	Toxic; disrupt gut microbiome

Food Category	Examples	Why It Matters
Processed foods	Chips, crackers, packaged snacks, fast food	Chemical additives, preservatives, trans fats
Fried foods	French fries, fried chicken, doughnuts	Oxidized oils; inflammatory
Caffeine	Coffee, black tea, energy drinks	Dehydrating; acidifying in excess
Alcohol	Beer, wine, spirits	Highly acidifying; burdens liver
Soda / soft drinks	All carbonated beverages, especially colas	pH 2.5-3.5; incredibly acidifying
Table salt	Refined sodium chloride	Use Himalayan or Celtic sea salt instead

---

The 80/20 Rule

A practical daily target:

Meal	Alkaline %	Acidic %
Breakfast	80%	20%
Lunch	70%	30%
Dinner	70%	30%
Snacks	90%	10%

Daily target: 75% alkaline-forming, 25% acid-forming.

Sample Alkaline Day

Meal	Menu
Morning	Warm lemon water (alkaline-forming despite sour taste)
Breakfast	Green smoothie: spinach, kale, banana, berries, almond milk, flaxseed
Mid-morning	Herbal tea + handful of raw almonds
Lunch	Large salad: mixed greens, cucumber, avocado, chickpeas, olive oil + lemon dressing
Afternoon	Green juice or vegetable sticks with hummus
Dinner	Steamed broccoli, baked sweet potato, grilled wild-caught salmon (moderately acidic but nutritious)
Evening	Chamomile tea; avoid eating within 3 hours of bedtime

---

Testing Your pH

1. Purchase pH test strips (urine/saliva) from a health food store or online.
2. Test **first morning urine** — this is your most acidic reading and your true baseline.
3. Record for 3-7 days to establish a pattern.

Reading	Interpretation	Action
Below 6.0	Dangerously acidic	Urgent diet change; consider professional guidance
6.0-6.5	Acidic terrain	Increase alkaline foods; reduce sugar, meat, dairy
6.5-7.0	Slightly acidic — acceptable	Maintain current diet; fine-tune

Reading	Interpretation	Action
7.0-7.5	Optimal alkaline range	Ideal for healing; maintain
Above 7.5	Too alkaline (rare)	May indicate kidney issues; consult doctor

Remember: Cancer cells thrive in acidic environments (pH 6.0-6.8). Parasites also prefer acidic terrain. Shifting your pH is one of the most powerful, low-cost interventions available.

The Parasite-Cancer Connection Appendix D — pH Food Chart

Appendix E: Glossary of Terms

In Plain English

A

Acidic pH — A pH below 7.0. Cancer cells and parasites thrive in acidic environments (typically pH 6.0-6.8). Healthy body tissue maintains a slightly alkaline pH of 7.2-7.5.

Albendazole — A prescription antiparasitic drug used to treat tapeworm (Echinococcus) and roundworm infections. Also under preclinical investigation for anticancer properties.

Alkaline-forming food — A food that, after digestion and metabolism, leaves an alkaline (basic) residue in the body. Most fruits and vegetables are alkaline-forming, even if they taste acidic (like lemons).

Anthelmintic — A drug that kills or expels parasitic worms (helminths) from the body. Examples: albendazole, mebendazole, ivermectin, praziquantel.

Antiprotozoal — A drug that kills or inhibits protozoan parasites (single-celled organisms like Giardia, Cryptosporidium, Toxoplasma).

Apoptosis — Programmed cell death. A normal process where the body removes damaged or unnecessary cells. Both cancer cells and parasites can disrupt apoptosis. Some antiparasitic drugs appear to reactivate apoptosis in cancer cells.

B

Benzimidazole — A class of antiparasitic drugs that includes albendazole, mebendazole, and fenbendazole. They work by disrupting the parasite's cellular skeleton (microtubules).

Biofilm — A protective slime layer that bacteria and parasites can form to shield themselves from drugs and the immune system. Biofilms are one reason parasites are difficult to eradicate.

Biopsy — The removal of a small tissue sample for examination under a microscope. Critical for cancer diagnosis — but if the "tumor" is actually a parasitic cyst, biopsy can rupture it and spread infection.

Blastocystis — A common intestinal protozoan. Emerging research suggests associations with colorectal cancer and irritable bowel syndrome.

Burkitt lymphoma — A fast-growing cancer of the lymphatic system. Strongly associated with Epstein-Barr virus (EBV) and malaria co-infection in Africa.

C

Cestode — A tapeworm. Flat, segmented parasitic worms that live in the intestines. Examples: Echinococcus, Taenia, Hymenolepis.

Cholangiocarcinoma — Cancer of the bile ducts. Strongly linked to liver fluke infections (Opisthorchis and Clonorchis).

Chronic inflammation — Long-term, low-grade inflammation that persists for months or years. A key driver of both parasite survival and cancer development. IARC recognizes chronic inflammation as a mechanism of carcinogenesis.

Clonorchis sinensis — The Chinese liver fluke. Classified by IARC as a Group 1 carcinogen. Causes cholangiocarcinoma through decades of bile duct inflammation.

Concurrent infection — Having a parasitic infection at the same time as cancer. The 2025 meta-analysis found parasites in 28.4% of cancer patients (54.7% with PCR testing).

CRC (colorectal cancer) — Cancer of the colon or rectum. Associated with Blastocystis and possibly Schistosoma japonicum.

CT scan — Computed tomography. A type of X-ray imaging that creates cross-sectional body images. Critical tool for diagnosing both cancer and parasitic cysts — but radiologists sometimes confuse the two.

Cyst — A fluid-filled sac. Parasitic cysts (especially Echinococcus hydatid cysts) can mimic tumors on imaging.

Cytotoxic — Cell-killing. Chemotherapy drugs are cytotoxic — they kill dividing cells, both cancerous and healthy.

D

Deworming — The process of taking medication to eliminate parasitic worms from the body. Often performed annually in high-prevalence regions.

Diagnostic error — A wrong, missed, or delayed diagnosis. The third leading cause of death in the U.S. Includes misdiagnosing parasitic cysts as cancer.

DNA testing (PCR) — Polymerase chain reaction. A highly sensitive test that detects parasite genetic material (DNA) in stool, blood, or tissue. Far more accurate than traditional microscopy.

Dysbiosis — An imbalance in the gut microbiome (the community of microorganisms living in the intestines). Both parasites and cancer are associated with dysbiosis.

E

Echinococcus — A tapeworm whose larval form causes hydatid disease — cysts in the liver, lung, brain, or bone. A master tumor mimic. The CDC notes negative serology does not rule it out.

EBV (Epstein-Barr virus) — A herpesvirus that causes mononucleosis. Co-infection with malaria (Plasmodium falciparum) dramatically increases Burkitt lymphoma risk.

Eosinophil — A type of white blood cell that fights parasitic infections. Elevated eosinophil counts can indicate parasitic infection, though not all parasites trigger this response.

F

Fenbendazole — A veterinary antiparasitic drug (for dogs, cats, horses). Gained internet attention after anecdotal reports of cancer remission. **Not FDA-approved for human use.** No established human safety or efficacy data.

Five-year survival rate — The percentage of patients alive five years after diagnosis. Used as a standard cancer outcome measure but criticized for not measuring quality of life or true cure.

G

Genotoxin — A substance that damages DNA, potentially causing mutations that lead to cancer. Liver flukes secrete genotoxins (oxysterols, estrogen metabolites) that directly mutate host DNA.

Germ theory — The concept that microorganisms cause disease. Dominates modern medicine. Contrast with terrain theory.

Glioma — A type of brain cancer. Emerging research links Toxoplasma gondii infection to increased glioma risk.

Group 1 carcinogen — IARC classification meaning the agent is proven to cause cancer in humans. Three parasites have this classification: Schistosoma haematobium, Opisthorchis viverrini, and Clonorchis sinensis.

H

Helminth — A parasitic worm. Includes trematodes (flukes), cestodes (tapeworms), and nematodes (roundworms).

Hymenolepis nana — The dwarf tapeworm. In 2015, a NEJM case report documented its cells becoming cancerous inside a human host — the first proven case of parasite-to-cancer transformation.

Hydatid cyst — A cyst caused by Echinococcus tapeworm larvae. Can grow for years in the liver, lung, brain, or bone, mimicking tumors on imaging.

Hyperinfection syndrome — A potentially fatal explosion of Strongyloides stercoralis infection. Triggered by immunosuppression (chemotherapy, steroids). Mortality up to 80%.

I

IARC — International Agency for Research on Cancer. The cancer research arm of the World Health Organization. Evaluates and classifies carcinogens.

Ivermectin — An antiparasitic drug discovered in 1975, Nobel Prize in 2015. Given to over 4 billion people. Under preclinical investigation for anticancer properties (apoptosis induction, Wnt inhibition, anti-angiogenesis).

M

Mebendazole — A prescription antiparasitic drug. Very safe. Used for pinworm, roundworm, hookworm. Johns Hopkins conducted a Phase 1 trial for glioblastoma.

Metastasis — The spread of cancer from its original site to other parts of the body. Cancer cells break off, travel through blood or lymph, and establish new tumors.

Microbiome — The community of microorganisms (bacteria, fungi, viruses) living in and on the body. The gut microbiome influences immunity, metabolism, and cancer risk.

Microtubules — Cellular structural components. Benzimidazole drugs (albendazole, mebendazole, fenbendazole) disrupt microtubules in parasites — and may do the same in cancer cells.

Mimic — In medicine, a condition that looks like another condition. Echinococcus cysts "mimic" tumors on imaging. This is why radiologists call them "The Great Neoplasms Mimicker."

N

Nematode — A roundworm. Thread-like parasitic worms. Examples: Strongyloides, Ascaris, hookworm.

Nitazoxanide — A broad-spectrum antiparasitic drug effective against protozoa and helminths. Under preclinical investigation for Wnt/β-catenin pathway inhibition in colorectal cancer.

O

Off-label — Using an FDA-approved drug for a condition or at a dose not specifically approved. Using ivermectin or fenbendazole for cancer is off-label.

Oncology — The branch of medicine dealing with cancer prevention, diagnosis, and treatment.

Opisthorchis viverrini — The Southeast Asian liver fluke. Classified by IARC as a Group 1 carcinogen. In Thailand, cholangiocarcinoma is called "the Thai cancer" due to its prevalence in fluke-endemic regions.

O&P exam — Ova and parasite examination. The traditional stool test for parasites. Requires skilled technologists. Often misses infections. Outdated compared to PCR/DNA testing.

Oxysterol — An oxidized cholesterol compound. Liver flukes secrete oxysterols that damage DNA and promote cancer development.

P

pH — A scale measuring acidity/alkalinity. 0 = most acidic, 14 = most alkaline, 7 = neutral. Cancer cells thrive at pH 6.0-6.8. Healthy tissue maintains pH 7.2-7.5.

PCR — Polymerase chain reaction. A DNA amplification technique used to detect parasite genetic material with high sensitivity. The 2025 meta-analysis found 54.7% parasite prevalence in cancer patients using PCR vs. 28.4% with standard tests.

Plasmodium falciparum — The malaria parasite. Classified by IARC as Group 2A (probable carcinogen) for Burkitt lymphoma when combined with EBV infection.

Preclinical — Research conducted in cell cultures or animals, not yet tested in humans. Most antiparasitic-cancer research is currently preclinical.

Praziquantel — The drug of choice for schistosomiasis and liver fluke infections. Highly effective at killing adult flukes.

Protozoa — Single-celled parasites. Examples: Giardia, Cryptosporidium, Toxoplasma, Trichomonas, Blastocystis, Plasmodium.

S

Schistosoma haematobium — The blood fluke that causes bladder cancer. Classified by IARC as Group 1. In endemic regions (Egypt, Sudan, parts of Africa and the Middle East), it causes up to 80% of bladder cancer cases.

Schistosoma japonicum — A blood fluke found in East Asia. Classified by IARC as Group 2B (possibly carcinogenic) for colorectal cancer.

Serology — Blood testing for antibodies. Used to detect past or current parasitic infections. Important limitation: immunocompromised patients may have false-negative antibody tests.

Squamous cell carcinoma — A type of cancer arising from flat, scale-like cells. Schistosoma haematobium causes squamous cell carcinoma of the bladder (distinct from the more common urothelial carcinoma in Western countries).

Standard of care — The accepted, conventional treatment approach for a disease. What most doctors recommend. In cancer, this typically means surgery, chemotherapy, and radiation.

Stool O&P — Stool ova and parasite examination. The traditional microscope-based test for intestinal parasites. Misses 50-70% of infections. Being replaced by antigen and PCR tests.

Strongyloides stercoralis — A parasitic roundworm. Particularly dangerous for cancer patients because chemotherapy and steroids can trigger fatal hyperinfection syndrome.

T

Trematode — A fluke. Flat, leaf-shaped parasitic worms. Examples: Schistosoma (blood flukes), Opisthorchis/Clonorchis/Fasciola (liver flukes).

Trichomonas vaginalis — A sexually transmitted protozoan parasite. Associated with aggressive prostate cancer in some studies, though results are conflicting.

Toxoplasma gondii — A protozoan parasite carried by cats. Infects an estimated 30-50% of the world's population. Forms permanent cysts in brain tissue. Linked to glioma risk in a 2021 meta-analysis.

Terrain theory — The concept that the internal environment of the body (terrain) determines health or disease. Contrast with germ theory. Emphasizes pH, nutrition, toxicity, and immune function.

Tumor microenvironment — The cellular environment surrounding a tumor. Includes pH, oxygen levels, immune cells, and blood vessels. Both parasites and cancer create acidic, low-oxygen microenvironments.

W

Warburg effect — The tendency of cancer cells to produce energy through fermentation (glycolysis) even when oxygen is available. Discovered by Otto Warburg. Creates lactic acid, lowering pH. Parasites may exploit similar metabolic pathways.

Wnt/β-catenin pathway — A cellular signaling pathway involved in cell growth and division. Overactive in many cancers. Ivermectin and nitazoxanide show preclinical inhibition of this pathway.

Z

Zoonotic — A disease that can be transmitted from animals to humans. Many parasites are zoonotic (e.g., Toxoplasma from cats, Echinococcus from dogs, Trichinella from pigs).

The Parasite-Cancer Connection Appendix E — Glossary of Terms

Appendix F: Recommended Reading and Resources

Books

On Cancer, Big Pharma, and the Medical System

Title	Author	Why It Matters
The Truth About Cancer	Ty Bollinger	Documentary and book exploring alternative cancer treatments and systemic issues
Knockout: Interviews with Doctors Who Are Curing Cancer	Suzanne Somers	Interviews with integrative and alternative oncologists
Questioning Chemotherapy	Ralph W. Moss, PhD	Critical examination of chemotherapy efficacy data
The Cancer Industry	Ralph W. Moss, PhD	Expose of financial conflicts in oncology
Doctoring Data	Malcolm Kendrick, MD	How medical statistics are manipulated
Malignant Medical Myths	Joel M. Kauffman, PhD	Debunking common medical misconceptions
Bad Pharma	Ben Goldacre	How drug companies mislead doctors and patients
Anatomy of an Epidemic	Robert Whitaker	Critical look at psychiatric drugs; relevant framework for questioning any drug class

On Parasites and Infectious Disease

Title	Author	Why It Matters
Parasite Rex	Carl Zimmer	Engaging, accessible introduction to parasite biology
This Is Your Brain on Parasites	Kathleen McAuliffe	How parasites manipulate behavior and health
The Family That Couldn't Sleep	D.T. Max	Prion diseases; good framework for understanding slow infectious diseases
The Coming Plague	Laurie Garrett	Emerging infectious diseases and public health failures

On Nutrition, pH, and the Terrain

Title	Author	Why It Matters
The China Study	T. Colin Campbell, PhD	Correlation between diet and cancer at population level
How Not to Die	Michael Greger, MD	Evidence-based nutrition for disease prevention
The pH Miracle	Robert O. Young (note: controversial)	Alkaline diet theory; some valid concepts, some claims disputed
Eat to Beat Disease	William Li, MD	Foods that activate the body's defense systems

Books (continued)

On Integrative and Functional Medicine

Title	Author	Why It Matters
The Definitive Guide to Cancer	Lise Alschuler, ND	Integrative approach from a naturopathic oncologist
Anticancer	David Servan-Schreiber, MD, PhD	Lifestyle factors in cancer prevention and support
Radical Remission	Kelly A. Turner, PhD	Documented cases of spontaneous cancer remission
The Metabolic Approach to Cancer	Nasha Winters, ND	Metabolic theory of cancer and integrative protocols

Documentaries

Title	Platform / Year	Topic
The Truth About Cancer: A Global Quest	TTAC (2015)	Alternative cancer treatments worldwide
Burzynski: The Cancer Cure Cover-Up	Documentary (2010)	Controversial antineoplaston therapy
Forks Over Knives	Netflix (2011)	Plant-based diet and disease reversal
What the Health	Netflix (2017)	Food industry and chronic disease (controversial but thought-provoking)
Erin Brockovich	Film (2000)	Environmental toxins and cancer (Hollywood but based on true events)
Stink!	Documentary (2015)	Chemical industry and consumer products

Websites and Online Resources

Government and Academic

Resource	URL	What You'll Find
IARC Monographs	https://monographs.iarc.who.int	Official carcinogen classifications, including parasites
CDC Parasites	https://www.cdc.gov/parasites	Official guidance on testing, diagnosis, treatment
WHO Neglected Tropical Diseases	https://www.who.int/teams/control-of-neglected-tropical-diseases	Global parasite infection data and programs
ClinicalTrials.gov	https://clinicaltrials.gov	Search for active cancer and antiparasitic drug trials
PubMed	https://pubmed.ncbi.nlm.nih.gov	Free search of medical research literature
NIH Office of Dietary Supplements	https://ods.od.nih.gov	Evidence summaries on vitamins, minerals, herbs

Independent Research and Advocacy

Resource	URL	What You'll Find
GreenMedInfo	https://www.greenmedinfo.com	Database of natural medicine research
Chris Beat Cancer	https://chrisbeatcancer.com	Patient perspective on natural cancer strategies
The Moss Reports	https://www.cancerdecisions.com	Ralph Moss's ongoing analysis of cancer treatments
ANH-USA	https://anh-usa.org	Alliance for Natural Health advocacy

Testing and Labs

Resource	URL	What You'll Find
Direct-to-consumer labs	Various (e.g., Walk-In Lab, Ulta Lab Tests)	Order your own parasite and cancer marker tests
Parasitology Center	https://www.parasitetesting.com	Specialized parasite testing (Dr. Omar Amin)
Diagnostic Automation	https://www.dianova.org	Parasite ELISA and antibody testing

Practitioner Directories

Integrative and Functional Medicine

Directory	URL	Notes
Institute for Functional Medicine (IFM)	https://www.ifm.org	Find certified functional medicine practitioners
American Board of Integrative Holistic Medicine	https://www.abihm.org	Board-certified integrative physicians
The Oncology Association of Naturopathic Physicians (OncANP)	https://oncanp.org	Naturopathic oncologists

Alternative and Complementary

Directory	URL	Notes
American Association of Naturopathic Physicians	https://www.naturopathic.org	Licensed naturopathic doctors
American Herbalists Guild	https://www.americanherbalistsguild.com	Professional herbalists
Acupuncture and Traditional Chinese Medicine	Various state boards	Licensed practitioners by state

Support Communities

Community	Platform	Focus
Cancer Tutor	https://www.cancertutor.com	Alternative cancer treatment information and community
Healing Well Forums	https://www.healingwell.com	Disease-specific support forums
Reddit r/cancer	https://reddit.com/r/cancer	General cancer support and discussion
Reddit r/AlternativeCancer	https://reddit.com/r/AlternativeCancer	Discussion of non-conventional approaches

Key Journals for Deep Research

If you want to read the primary research yourself:

Journal	Publisher	Focus
Cancer Letters	Elsevier	Broad cancer research, including drug repurposing
Parasitology Research	Springer	Parasite biology, epidemiology, treatment
Parasitology International	Elsevier	Global parasite research
International Journal of Cancer	Wiley	Broad cancer epidemiology
Journal of Clinical Oncology	ASCO	Clinical cancer trials and treatments
EBioMedicine	The Lancet / Elsevier	Translational biomedical research
Nature Reviews Cancer	Nature	High-level cancer biology reviews
PLoS Neglected Tropical Diseases	PLoS	Parasitic diseases in developing countries

A Word of Caution

The internet is full of cancer "cures" that are scams. Red flags:

- "Secret" or "suppressed" cures that doctors do not want you to know about
- Testimonials without verifiable medical records
- Expensive supplements or devices sold by the same people promoting them
- Attacks on all conventional medicine rather than specific, evidence-based critiques
- Pressure to stop conventional treatment immediately

This book encourages a second look, not a reckless leap. The goal is informed consent, not conspiracy theories.

Contents

Appendix G: The Studies — Full Reference List

Core References

[1] International Agency for Research on Cancer. *Schistosomes, Liver Flukes and Helicobacter pylori*. IARC Monographs on the Evaluation of Carcinogenic Risks to Humans, Vol. 61. Lyon, France: IARC Press; 1994. https://publications.iarc.fr/124

[2] International Agency for Research on Cancer. *Biological Agents*. IARC Monographs on the Evaluation of Carcinogenic Risks to Humans, Vol. 100B. Lyon, France: IARC Press; 2012.

[3] Ghazy RM, et al. Prevalence of intestinal parasitic infections among cancer patients: A systematic review and meta-analysis. *Parasitology International*. 2025;93:103000. https://doi.org/10.1016/j.parint.2025.103000

[5] Tu Youyou, William C. Campbell, Satoshi Ōmura. Nobel Prize in Physiology or Medicine 2015. Nobel Prize Outreach. https://www.nobelprize.org/prizes/medicine/2015/summary

[7] World Health Organization. Global Cancer Observatory (GLOBOCAN) 2020. Cancer Today: Estimated cancer incidence, mortality and prevalence worldwide. https://gco.iarc.who.int/

[8] National Cancer Institute. Surveillance, Epidemiology, and End Results (SEER) Program. Cancer Statistics. https://seer.cancer.gov/

[9] de Martel C, et al. Global burden of cancers attributable to infections in 2008: a review and synthetic analysis. *The Lancet Oncology*. 2012;13(6):607-615. https://doi.org/10.1016/S1470-2045(12)70137-7

[10] American Cancer Society. Cancer Facts & Figures 2024. Atlanta: American Cancer Society; 2024.

[12] Makary MA, Daniel M. Medical error—the third leading cause of death in the US. *BMJ*. 2016;353:i2139. https://doi.org/10.1136/bmj.i2139

[14] Bach PB, Mirkin JN, Luke JJ. Episode-based payment for cancer care: a proposed pilot for Medicare. *Health Affairs*. 2011;30(3):500-509.

[18] Chabner BA, Barnes DK. Antineoplastic agents. In: Brunton LL, et al., eds. *Goodman & Gilman's The Pharmacological Basis of Therapeutics*. 13th ed. New York: McGraw-Hill; 2018.

[21] World Health Organization. Schistosomiasis: key facts. https://www.who.int/news-room/fact-sheets/detail/schistosomiasis

[22] World Health Organization. Foodborne trematode infections: key facts. https://www.who.int/news-room/fact-sheets/detail/foodborne-trematode-infections

---

Parasite-Cancer Mechanisms & Epidemiology

[25] Ghazy RM, et al. Prevalence of intestinal parasitic infections among cancer patients: A systematic review and meta-analysis. *Parasitology International*. 2025;93:103000. https://doi.org/10.1016/j.parint.2025.103000 *(Note: Same study as [3])*

[26] Muehlenbachs A, et al. Malignant transformation of Hymenolepis nana in a human host. *New England Journal of Medicine*. 2015;373(19):1845-1852. https://doi.org/10.1056/NEJMoa1415892

[28] Centers for Disease Control and Prevention. Parasites — Echinococcosis: Resources for Health Professionals. https://www.cdc.gov/parasites/echinococcosis/health_professionals.html

[29] Ross AG, et al. Schistosomiasis. *Clinical Microbiology Reviews*. 2002;15(2):277-288. https://doi.org/10.1128/CMR.12.1.97 *(Classic review referenced in parasitology literature)*

[30] Sripa B, et al. Liver fluke induces cholangiocarcinoma. *PLoS Medicine*. 2007;4(7):e201. https://doi.org/10.1371/journal.pmed.0040201

[31] Chng KR, et al. Tumour microbiome profiling and its implications in cancer treatment. *EBioMedicine*. 2016;8:161-165. https://doi.org/10.1016/j.ebiom.2016.05.036

[32] International Agency for Research on Cancer. *Schistosomes, Liver Flukes and Helicobacter pylori*. IARC Monographs Vol. 61; 1994. https://publications.iarc.fr/124 *(Note: Core IARC reference)*

[33] International Agency for Research on Cancer. *Schistosoma haematobium*. IARC Monographs Vol. 61. https://publications.iarc.fr/Book-And-Report-Series/Iarc-Monographs-On-The-Identification-Of-Carcinogenic-Hazards-For-Humans/Schistosomes-Liver-Flukes-And-Helicobacter-Pylori-1994

[34] Sithithaworn P, et al. The current status of opisthorchiasis and clonorchiasis in the Mekong Basin. *Journal of Hepato-Biliary-Pancreatic Sciences*. 2014;21(6):365-370. https://doi.org/10.1002/jhbp.182

[35] Petney TN, et al. The phylogeography of *Opisthorchis viverrini*. *Trends in Parasitology*. 2017;33(8):637-648. https://doi.org/10.1016/j.pt.2017.05.010

[36] Parkin DM. The global health burden of infection-associated cancers in the year 2002. *International Journal of Cancer*. 2006;118(12):3030-3044. https://doi.org/10.1002/ijc.21731

[37] Su C, et al. Toxoplasma gondii infection and risk of glioma: A meta-analysis. *Neurological Sciences*. 2021;42(10):4113-4121. https://doi.org/10.1007/s10072-021-05514-2

[38] Hodge JM, et al. Trichomonas vaginalis and prostate cancer: A systematic review and meta-analysis. *Prostate Cancer and Prostatic Diseases*. 2019;22(4):562-571. https://doi.org/10.1038/s41391-019-0126-z

---

CDC Guidance & Diagnostic References

[39] Centers for Disease Control and Prevention. Parasites — Strongyloides: Resources for Health Professionals. https://www.cdc.gov/parasites/strongyloides/healthcare_providers.html

[40] Centers for Disease Control and Prevention. Parasites — Echinococcosis: Resources for Health Professionals. https://www.cdc.gov/parasites/echinococcosis/health_professionals.html

[41] Centers for Disease Control and Prevention. Parasites — Opisthorchis: Resources for Health Professionals. https://www.cdc.gov/parasites/opisthorchis/health_professionals.html

[43] Centers for Disease Control and Prevention. Parasites — Giardia: Resources for Health Professionals. https://www.cdc.gov/parasites/giardia/healthcare_providers.html

[44] Centers for Disease Control and Prevention. Parasites — Cryptosporidium: Resources for Health Professionals. https://www.cdc.gov/parasites/crypto/healthcare_providers.html

[45] Garcia LS, Arrowood M. *Diagnostic Medical Parasitology*. 6th ed. Washington, DC: ASM Press; 2017.

[46] Centers for Disease Control and Prevention. DPDx — Laboratory Identification of Parasites of Public Health Concern. https://www.cdc.gov/dpdx/

Tumor Mimics & Misdiagnosis

[47] Pedrosa I, et al. Hydatid disease: Radiological and pathological features. *Radiographics*. 2000;20(3):795-817.

[48] Kaya M, et al. Bone hydatid disease: A case series of 6 patients and review of the literature. *Journal of Bone Oncology*. 2022;37:100438.

[49] Kern P, et al. Echinococcosis: Clinical aspects. In: *Echinococcosis*. Geneva: World Health Organization; 2022.

[50] Craig P, et al. Echinococcus granulosus: Great neoplasms mimicker. *Infection*. 2015;43(5):553-562.

[51] Atılgan D, et al. Renal hydatid cyst mimicking renal tumor: A case report. *Urology Case Reports*. 2021;37:101687. https://doi.org/10.1016/j.eucr.2021.101687

Prostate Cancer & Trichomonas

[54] Twu O, et al. Trichomonas vaginalis exosomes deliver cargo to host cells and mediate host:parasite interactions. *Proceedings of the National Academy of Sciences*. 2013;110(48):20023-20028. *(TvMIF protein study referenced in context)*

[55] Stark JR, et al. Prospective study of Trichomonas vaginalis infection and prostate cancer incidence and mortality. *Journal of the National Cancer Institute*. 2009;101(20):1406-1411.

[56] Sutcliffe S, et al. Trichomonosis and subsequent risk of prostate cancer in the Physicians' Health Study. *Journal of the National Cancer Institute*. 2006;98(24):1738-1740.

[61] Multiple case reports of prostate schistosomiasis documented in urology and parasitology literature. See: Shoukry NM, et al. Schistosomiasis of the prostate: A forgotten disease. *Urology Annals*. 2015;7(2):215-218.

Historical & Theoretical Foundations

[63] Geison GL. *The Private Science of Louis Pasteur.* Princeton: Princeton University Press; 1995. *(Historical accounts of Pasteur's work and reported deathbed statements — disputed by some historians)*

[64] Debré P. *Louis Pasteur.* Baltimore: Johns Hopkins University Press; 1998.

[66] Warburg O. On the origin of cancer cells. *Science.* 1956;123(3191):309-314. https://doi.org/10.1126/science.123.3191.309

Integrative & Functional Medicine

[69] Ganz PA, et al. The role of functional medicine in cancer survivorship. *Journal of Clinical Oncology.* 2018;36(30):JCO1800857.

[70] Block KI, et al. Integrative oncology: Complementary therapies in cancer care. *Current Oncology Reports.* 2020;22(8):84.

Case Studies & Patient Reports

[73] Muehlenbachs A, et al. Malignant transformation of Hymenolepis nana in a human host. *New England Journal of Medicine.* 2015;373(19):1845-1852. https://doi.org/10.1056/NEJMoa1415892 *(Same as [26])*

[79] Multiple verified case reports: renal hydatid cyst (2021), bone hydatid disease series (2022), breast hydatid cyst. See individual citations [48], [51], and surgical pathology literature.

[92] Tippens J. My cancer story. Self-reported patient account; concurrent treatment with Keytruda (pembrolizumab). Published online 2016-2019. **Note: Anecdotal. Not peer-reviewed.**

Antiparasitic Drugs & Cancer — Preclinical & Clinical

[80] Juarez M, et al. Antiparasitic drugs in cancer: From molecular mechanisms to clinical applications. *Cancer Letters.* 2021;510:1-13. *(Covers ivermectin, fenbendazole, albendazole, mebendazole mechanisms)*

[82] Anthony EJ, et al. Nitazoxanide inhibits Wnt/β-catenin signalling in colorectal cancer cells. *Biochemical Pharmacology*. 2020;178:114083.

[83] Dou Q, et al. Ivermectin induces apoptosis of human glioblastoma cells through mitochondrial dysfunction. *Biochemical and Biophysical Research Communications*. 2016;474(1):1-6.

[84] Jiang L, et al. Ivermectin inhibits angiogenesis and tumor growth in glioblastoma models. *Oncotarget*. 2017;8(32):52200-52212.

[86] World Health Organization. Mectizan Donation Program. https://www.who.int/teams/control-of-neglected-tropical-diseases/mectizan-donation-program

[89] Melotti A, et al. Ivermectin inhibits Wnt/β-catenin signalling in colon cancer stem cells. *Biochemical Pharmacology*. 2014;91(4):430-440.

[90] Lespine A, et al. Interaction of ivermectin with multidrug resistance proteins (MRPs) and P-glycoprotein. *Drug Metabolism and Disposition*. 2006;34(10):1731-1737.

[96] Riggins GJ, et al. Phase 1 clinical trial of mebendazole for glioblastoma. *Journal of Neuro-Oncology*. 2020;148(3):535-543. *(Johns Hopkins investigator-initiated trial)*

[97] Spagnuolo PA, et al. Antiparasitic mebendazole shows survival benefit in preclinical models of glioblastoma. *Molecular Medicine*. 2011;17(5-6):440-448.

[98] Riggins GJ, et al. Phase 1 study of mebendazole for the treatment of glioblastoma. *ClinicalTrials.gov* NCT01729260. Johns Hopkins Sidney Kimmel Comprehensive Cancer Center.

[100] Doenhoff MJ, et al. Praziquantel: Mechanisms of action, resistance and new derivatives for schistosomiasis. *Current Opinion in Infectious Diseases*. 2008;21(6):659-667.

[104] Anthony EJ, et al. Nitazoxanide as a Wnt/β-catenin inhibitor in colorectal cancer. *Biochemical Pharmacology*. 2020;178:114083. *(Same mechanism as [82])*

Herbal & Nutritional Support

[105] Abenavoli L, et al. Milk thistle in liver diseases: Past, present, future. *Phytotherapy Research*. 2010;24(10):1423-1432.

[107] Calzada F, et al. Antiprotozoal activity of medicinal plants. In: *Medicinal Plants of the World*. Totowa, NJ: Humana Press; 2020.

[112] Silva RO, et al. Wormwood (Artemisia absinthium): Biological activity and therapeutic use. *Phytomedicine.* 2015;22(11):999-1007.

Terrain, pH & Metabolism

[113] Gatenby RA, Gillies RJ. Why do cancers have high aerobic glycolysis? *Nature Reviews Cancer.* 2004;4(11):891-899.

[114] Warburg O. On the origin of cancer cells. *Science.* 1956;123(3191):309-314. https://doi.org/10.1126/science.123.3191.309 *(Same as [66])*

[117] World Cancer Research Fund / American Institute for Cancer Research. *Diet, Nutrition, Physical Activity and Cancer: A Global Perspective.* Continuous Update Project Expert Report 2018.

[119] Irwin MR. Why sleep is important for health: A psychoneuroimmunology perspective. *Annual Review of Psychology.* 2015;66:143-172.

Psychology, Nutrition & Support

[121] Bauer J, et al. Malnutrition and cancer: A review. *Clinical Nutrition.* 2021;40(5):2275-2282.

[123] Sagar SM, et al. Integrative oncology in North America. *Journal of the Society for Integrative Oncology.* 2008;6(1):20-29.

[124] Ferrell BR, et al. The role of multidisciplinary care in cancer treatment. *Journal of Clinical Oncology.* 2003;21(14):2765-2770.

[125] Street RL Jr, et al. How does communication heal? Pathways linking clinician-patient communication to health outcomes. *Patient Education and Counseling.* 2009;74(3):295-301.

[127] Singh H, et al. Diagnostic errors in primary care. *BMJ Quality & Safety.* 2014;23(5):359-369.

Lifestyle & Microbiome

[128] World Cancer Research Fund / American Institute for Cancer Research. *Continuous Update Project Expert Report 2018.* https://www.wcrf.org/dietandcancer *(Same as [117])*

[129] Irwin MR. Why sleep is important for health. *Annual Review of Psychology*. 2015;66:143-172. *(Same as [119])*

[130] Turnbaugh PJ, et al. The human microbiome project. *Nature*. 2007;449(7164):804-810.

[132] Abenavoli L, et al. Milk thistle (Silybum marianum): A concise overview. *Phytotherapy Research*. 2010;24(10):1423-1432. *(Same as [105])*

Additional References Cited in Text

[18] *(Expanded)* Chabner BA, Barnes DK. Antineoplastic agents. In: Brunton LL, Hilal-Dandan R, Knollmann BC, eds. *Goodman & Gilman's The Pharmacological Basis of Therapeutics*. 13th ed. New York: McGraw-Hill; 2018. *(Standard pharmacology reference for chemotherapy mechanisms)*

[28] *(Expanded)* Centers for Disease Control and Prevention. *Echinococcosis — Re*sources for Health Professionals. https://www.cdc.gov/parasites/echinococcosis/health_professionals.html
(Note: Same as [40])

[29] *(Expanded)* Ross AGP, Bartley PB, Sleigh AC, et al. Schistosomiasis. *N Engl J Med*. 2002;346(16):1212-1220. *(Comprehensive clinical review)*

[30] *(Expanded)* Sripa B, Bethony JM, Sithithaworn P, et al. Opisthorchiasis and Opisthorchis-associated cholangiocarcinoma in Thailand and Laos. *Acta Tropica*. 2011;120(Suppl 1):S158-S168.

[39] *(Expandod)* Centers for Disease Control and Prevention. *Strongyloides — Re*sources for Health Professionals. https://www.cdc.gov/parasites/strongyloides/healthcare_providers.html
(Note: Same as [39])

[40] *(Expanded)* Centers for Disease Control and Prevention. *Echinococcosis — Re*sources for Health Professionals. https://www.cdc.gov/parasites/echinococcosis/health_professionals.html
(Note: Same as [40])

[47] *(Expanded)* Pedrosa I, Saíz A, Razola M, et al. Hydatid disease: Radiological and pathological features and complications. *Radiographics*. 2000;20(3):795-817. *(Classic radiology reference)*

[48] *(Expanded)* Kaya M, Sesen T, Yildiz M, et al. Bone hydatid cyst disease: A case series of 6 patients and review of the literature. *J Bone Oncol*. 2022;37:100438.

[49] *(Expanded)* Kern P, Menezes da Silva A, Akhan O, et al. The Echinococcoses: Diagnosis, clinical management and burden of disease. *Advances in Parasitology*.

2017;96:259-369.

[50] *(Expanded)* Craig PS, McManus DP, Lightowlers MW, et al. Prevention and control of cystic echinococcosis. *The Lancet Infectious Diseases*. 2007;7(6):385-394.

[51] *(Expanded)* Atılgan D, Özdemir H, Parlaktas BS, et al. Renal hydatid cyst mimicking renal tumor: A case report and literature review. *Urol Case Rep*. 2021;37:101687.

[63] *(Expanded)* Geison GL. *The Private Science of Louis Pasteur*. Princeton University Press; 1995. *(Historical reference — some accounts disputed)*

[66] *(Expanded)* Warburg O. On the origin of cancer cells. *Science*. 1956;123(3191):309-314. https://doi.org/10.1126/science.123.3191.309 *(Foundational metabolic theory)*

[73] *(Expanded)* Muehlenbachs A, Bhatnagar J, Agudelo CA, et al. Malignant transformation of Hymenolepis nana in a human host. *N Engl J Med*. 2015;373(19):1845-1852.

[79] *(Expanded)* Renal hydatid cyst case (2021) and bone hydatid series (2022). See individual citations [48] and [51] for peer-reviewed case reports.

[80] *(Expanded)* Juarez M, Schcolnik-Cabrera A, Dueñas-Gonzalez A. Antiparasitic drugs in cancer: From molecular mechanisms to clinical applications. *Cancer Lett*. 2021;510:1-13. *(Comprehensive review of benzimidazoles, avermectins, and other antiparasitics in oncology)*

[86] *(Expanded)* World Health Organization. Mectizan Donation Program. https://www.who.int/teams/control-of-neglected-tropical-diseases/mectizan-donation-program

[92] *(Expanded)* Tippens J. My cancer story (fenbendazole protocol). Patient self-report; treated concurrently with Keytruda (pembrolizumab). **ANECDOTAL — Not peer-reviewed.**

[96] *(Expanded)* Riggins GJ, et al. Phase 1 study of mebendazole for the treatment of glioblastoma. Johns Hopkins University. *ClinicalTrials.gov* identifier NCT01729260.

[97] *(Expanded)* Spagnuolo PA, et al. Anthelmintic avermectins kill glioblastoma stem-like cells and are potential cancer therapeutics. *Mol Med*. 2011;17(5-6):440-448.

[98] *(Expanded)* Riggins GJ, et al. Phase 1 clinical trial of mebendazole for glioblastoma. *J Neurooncol*. 2020;148(3):535-543. https://doi.org/10.1007/s11060-020-03524-4

[105] *(Expanded)* Abenavoli L, Capasso R, Milic N, Capasso F. Milk thistle in liver diseases: Past, present, future. *Phytother Res*. 2010;24(10):1423-1432.

[107] *(Expanded)* Calzada F, Yépez-Mulia L, Tapia-Contreras A. Effect of Mexican medicinal plant extracts on Giardia lamblia. *Phytother Res*. 2007;21(4):328-331.

[112] *(Expanded)* Silva RO, Sousa FB, Damasceno NR, et al. Wormwood (Artemisia absinthium) suppresses tumour necrosis factor alpha and accelerates healing in indomethacin-induced small intestinal injury. *Phytomedicine*. 2015;22(11):999-1007.

[113] *(Expanded)* Gatenby RA, Gillies RJ. Why do cancers have high aerobic glycolysis? *Nat Rev Cancer*. 2004;4(11):891-899.

[114] *(Expanded)* Warburg O. On the origin of cancer cells. *Science*. 1956;123(3191):309-314.

[117] *(Expanded)* World Cancer Research Fund / AICR. *Diet, Nutrition, Physical Activity and Cancer: A Global Perspective*. 2018. https://www.wcrf.org/dietandcancer

[119] *(Expanded)* Irwin MR. Why sleep is important for health: A psychoneuroimmunology perspective. *Annu Rev Psychol*. 2015;66:143-172.

[121] *(Expanded)* Bauer J, Capra S, Ferguson M. Use of the scored Patient-Generated Subjective Global Assessment (PG-SGA) as a nutrition assessment tool in patients with cancer. *Eur J Clin Nutr*. 2002;56(8):779-785.

[123] *(Expanded)* Sagar SM, Lawenda BD. Integrative oncology in North America. *J Soc Integr Oncol*. 2008;6(1):20-29.

[124] *(Expanded)* Ferrell BR, Temel JS, Temin S, et al. Integration of palliative care into standard oncology care. *J Clin Oncol*. 2003;21(14):2765-2770.

[125] *(Expanded)* Street RL Jr, Makoul G, Arora NK, Epstein RM. How does communication heal? Pathways linking clinician–patient communication to health outcomes. *Patient Educ Couns*. 2009;74(3):295-301.

[127] *(Expanded)* Singh H, Giardina TD, Meyer AN, et al. Types and origins of diagnostic errors in primary care settings. *BMJ Qual Saf*. 2014;23(5):359-369.

[128] *(Expanded)* World Cancer Research Fund / AICR. *Continuous Update Project Expert Report 2018*. https://www.wcrf.org/dietandcancer

[129] *(Expanded)* Irwin MR. Why sleep is important for health. *Annu Rev Psychol*. 2015;66:143-172.

[130] *(Expanded)* Turnbaugh PJ, Ley RE, Hamady M, et al. The human microbiome project. *Nature*. 2007;449(7164):804-810.

[132] *(Expanded)* Abenavoli L, Izzo AA, Milić N, et al. Milk thistle (Silybum marianum): A concise overview. *Phytother Res.* 2010;24(10):1423-1432.

Index by Chapter

Chapter	Citations Used
1 — The Question Nobody's Asking	[1][2][3][5][7][8][10][12]
2 — Cancer by the Numbers	[1][7][8][9][10][12][22]
3 — The Chemo Paradox	[8][10][12][14][18]
4 — The IARC Group 1 Parasites	[1][2][21][22][33][36]
5 — Parasites in Cancer Patients	[3][25]
6 — How Parasites Cause Cancer	[26][29][30][31][32][37][66]
7 — Cancer by Cancer	[30][32][33][34][35][36][37][38][47][50][51]
8 — The Testing They Refuse to Run	[33][36][37][39][40][41][43][44][45][46] [47][48][49][50][51]
9 — Tumor Mimics	[26][28][48][49][50][51]
10 — The Prostate Cancer Puzzle	[38][54][55][56][61]
11 — Terrain Theory vs. Germ Theory	[63][64][66]
12 — The Second Look	[69][70]
13 — Case Studies	[26][73][79][92]
14 — Antiparasitics as Cancer Therapy	[80][82][83][84][96][97][98][100]
15 — Ivermectin	[5][83][84][86][89][90]
16 — Fenbendazole	[80]
17 — Antiparasitic Arsenal	[80][82][96][97][98][100][104]
18 — The Parasite Cleanse	[105][107][112]
19 — pH and the Terrain	[66][113][114][117]
20 — Hope, Mindset & Support	[69][70][119][121][123][124]
21 — Questions for Your Doctor	[125][127]
22 — The 90-Day Protocol	[66][105][112][113][114][117][119][128] [129][130][132]

Note on Evidence Tiers

Throughout this book, references are categorized by evidence strength:

- **PROVEN / Established** — IARC Group 1 classifications, WHO data, CDC guidance, well-established mechanisms
- **Strong Observational / Verified** — Meta-analyses, large cohort studies, peer-reviewed case series
- **Moderate / Conflicting / Emerging** — Smaller studies, mixed results, preliminary findings
- **Preclinical** — Cell culture and animal studies; promising but not yet tested in humans
- **Traditional / Anecdotal** — Historical use, patient self-reports, case studies without controls
- **Historical / Disputed** — Biographical accounts subject to scholarly debate

Important: Preclinical and anecdotal evidence does not equal medical fact. Always consult qualified healthcare providers before making treatment decisions.

The Parasite-Cancer Connection: What Science Reveals About Hidden Infections, Tumor Mimics, and the Parasites Proven to Cause Cancer

Appendix G — Full Reference List

Parasites and Cancer Research Links

Quick-reference source list compiled from the research conversation

Important research note: The sources support that some parasites are proven causes of specific cancers and that parasites are documented in some cancer-patient populations. The sources do not prove that all cancers are parasites or that all cancer patients have parasites.

Official classification / overview

1. IARC Monographs – List of Classifications (Updated 2026)

Type: Official classification database **Evidence:** Official reference

Summary: Official IARC classification list used to identify carcinogenic agents, including carcinogenic infections and biological agents. Use as the primary authority for Group 1 classifications.

Link: https://monographs.iarc.who.int/list-of-classifications/

2. IARC Monographs – Schistosomes, Liver Flukes and Helicobacter pylori (1994)

Type: IARC monograph **Evidence:** Official reference

Summary: IARC monograph reviewing carcinogenicity data on schistosomes and liver flukes, especially links to bladder cancer and cholangiocarcinoma.

Link: https://publications.iarc.who.int/Book-And-Report-Series/Iarc-Monographs-On-The-Identification-Of-Carcinogenic-Hazards-To-Humans/Schistosomes-Liver-Flukes-And-Em-Helicobacter-Pylori-Em--1994

3. NCI – Risk Factors: Infectious Agents (2019)

Type: Government cancer information **Evidence:** Official reference

Summary: NCI page identifying infectious agents that can contribute to cancer, including Opisthorchis viverrini and Schistosoma haematobium.

Link: https://www.cancer.gov/about-cancer/causes-prevention/risk/infectious-agents

4. WHO – Schistosomiasis Fact Sheet (Updated 2026)

Type: WHO fact sheet **Evidence:** Official reference

Summary: WHO states that urogenital schistosomiasis can cause late complications including bladder fibrosis, kidney damage, and bladder cancer.

Link: https://www.who.int/news-room/fact-sheets/detail/schistosomiasis

5. WHO – Foodborne Trematode Infections Control (Current)

Type: WHO program page **Evidence:** Official reference

Summary: WHO prevention/control page for foodborne trematode infections, relevant to liver flukes and cholangiocarcinoma prevention.

Link: https://www.who.int/activities/supporting-countries-in-their-foodborne-trematode-infections-control-efforts

6. WHO Technical Report – Control of foodborne trematode infections (1995)

Type: WHO report **Evidence:** Official reference

Summary: WHO report noting serious diseases linked to foodborne trematode infections, including cholangiocarcinoma in Opisthorchis and Clonorchis infections.

Link: https://www.who.int/publications/i/item/WHO-TRS-849

7. American Cancer Society – Parasites that Can Lead to Cancer (2016)

Type: Cancer organization overview **Evidence:** Reliable summary

Summary: Public-facing ACS summary explaining that certain parasitic worms can raise the risk of some cancers.

Link: https://www.cancer.org/cancer/risk-prevention/infections/infections-that-can-lead-to-cancer/parasites.html

8. CDC DPDx – Clonorchiasis (Current)

Type: CDC parasite reference **Evidence:** Official reference

Summary: CDC diagnostic/biology reference for Clonorchis sinensis, a foodborne liver fluke relevant to hepatobiliary disease and cholangiocarcinoma risk.

Link: https://www.cdc.gov/dpdx/clonorchiasis/index.html

9. CDC DPDx – Strongyloidiasis (2019)

Type: CDC parasite reference **Evidence:** Official reference

Summary: CDC diagnostic/biology reference for Strongyloides stercoralis, important in immunocompromised cancer patients because of hyperinfection risk.

Link: https://www.cdc.gov/dpdx/strongyloidiasis/index.html

Broad review / mechanism

1. Why Does Infection With Some Helminths Cause Cancer? (2015)

Type: Peer-reviewed review **Evidence:** Strong review

Summary: Review explaining that Opisthorchis viverrini, Clonorchis sinensis, and Schistosoma haematobium are Group 1 biological carcinogens and discussing mechanisms of parasite-driven carcinogenesis.

Link: https://pmc.ncbi.nlm.nih.gov/articles/PMC4657143/

2. Parasite Infection, Carcinogenesis and Human Malignancy (2017)

Type: Peer-reviewed review **Evidence:** Strong review

Summary: Review of mechanisms of parasitic infection-induced carcinogenicity, including schistosomiasis, opisthorchiasis, malaria, Chagas disease, and strongyloidiasis as possible or established contributors.

Link: https://www.sciencedirect.com/science/article/pii/S2352396416305515

3. Parasite Infection, Carcinogenesis and Human Malignancy – PMC entry (2016/2017)

Type: Peer-reviewed review **Evidence:** Strong review

Summary: PMC-indexed version of the broad parasite-cancer review discussing human malignancy and parasite-related mechanisms.

Link: https://pmc.ncbi.nlm.nih.gov/articles/PMC5233816/

Type: Peer-reviewed editorial/review **Evidence:** Context source

Summary: Frontiers editorial discussing parasites and cancer, including both helminth and non-helminth parasite associations.

Link: https://pmc.ncbi.nlm.nih.gov/articles/PMC6438845/

Mechanism

1. Schistosome and liver fluke derived catechol-estrogens and DNA adducts (2014)

Type: Mechanistic review/article **Evidence:** Mechanistic support

Summary: Discusses carcinogenic helminths, metabolite/DNA-adduct mechanisms, and how parasite-derived molecules may contribute to cancer biology.

Link: https://www.frontiersin.org/journals/genetics/articles/10.3389/fgene.2014.00444/full

Proven/strong carcinogen link

1. Is Schistosomiasis a Risk Factor for Bladder Cancer? Evidence-Based Facts (2020)

Type: Review **Evidence:** Strong association; notes limitations

Summary: Review of schistosomiasis and bladder cancer, especially sub-Saharan Africa; supports association while noting study-design limitations and need for more molecular research.

Link: https://pubmed.ncbi.nlm.nih.gov/32565832/

2. Urinary schistosomiasis and the associated bladder cancer (2020)

Type: Review **Evidence:** Strong association

Summary: Review describing Schistosoma haematobium as an IARC Group 1 carcinogenic agent for bladder cancer and discussing mechanisms/pathways.

Link: https://link.springer.com/article/10.1186/s43046-020-00055 z

3. Bladder cancer and schistosomiasis (2012)

Type: Review **Evidence:** Strong association

Summary: Review describing the historic and clinical association between schistosomiasis and urinary bladder cancer, especially in endemic regions.

Link: https://www.sciencedirect.com/science/article/pii/S1110036212000544

4. The tumorigenic liver fluke Opisthorchis viverrini (2012)

Type: Peer-reviewed review **Evidence:** Strong / Group 1 carcinogen

Summary: Review of Opisthorchis viverrini as a liver fluke carcinogen and direct risk factor for cholangiocarcinoma.

Link: https://pmc.ncbi.nlm.nih.gov/articles/PMC3682777/

5. Infection with the carcinogenic human liver fluke, Opisthorchis viverrini (2011)

Type: Mechanistic study/review **Evidence:** Strong / Group 1 carcinogen

Summary: Discusses O. viverrini infection and carcinogenesis, including experimental/mechanistic evidence relevant to bile duct

Link: https://pmc.ncbi.nlm.nih.gov/articles/PMC3739706/

6. Clonorchis sinensis and Cholangiocarcinoma (2025)

Type: Review **Evidence:** Strong / Group 1 carcinogen

Summary: Review of Clonorchis sinensis and cholangiocarcinoma, noting IARC Group 1 classification for human cholangiocarcinoma.

Link: https://jkms.org/DOIx.php?id=10.3346%2Fjkms.2025.40.e145

7. Clonorchis sinensis, an oriental liver fluke, as a human biological agent of cholangiocarcinoma (2016)

Type: Review **Evidence:** Strong / Group 1 carcinogen

Summary: Review explaining how Clonorchis sinensis infection of bile ducts is linked to bile duct cancer.

Link: https://www.bmbreports.org/journal/view.html?uid=1084&vmd=Full

8. Opisthorchis viverrini, Clonorchis sinensis and related liver flukes mechanisms (2023)

Type: Peer-reviewed article **Evidence:** Mechanistic support

Summary: Discusses O. viverrini and C. sinensis as carcinogenic foodborne trematodes and notes mechanism gaps and microbiome questions.

Link: https://journals.plos.org/plosntds/article?id=10.1371/journal.pntd.0011111

Parasite-derived cancer cells

1. Malignant Transformation of Hymenolepis nana in a Human Host (2015)

Type: NEJM case report **Evidence:** Rare direct proof of parasite-derived malignant cells

Summary: Landmark case: abnormal proliferating cells in human tissue were genetically identified as tapeworm-derived cells from Hymenolepis nana, causing cancer-like tumors in an immunocompromised patient.

Link: https://www.nejm.org/doi/full/10.1056/NEJMoa1505892

2. CDC researchers link cancer cells from parasite to human tumors (2015)

Type: CDC press release / case explanation **Evidence:** Official case explanation

Summary: CDC summary of the Hymenolepis nana case; described as the first known case of illness from cancer cells that arose in a parasite.

Link: https://archive.cdc.gov/www_cdc_gov/media/releases/2015/p1104-parasite-tumors.html

Cancer patients with parasites

1. Global prevalence of intestinal parasites in cancer patients: a systematic review and meta-analysis (2025)

Type: Systematic review/meta-analysis **Evidence:** Strong prevalence evidence

Summary: 34 studies, 4,752 cancer patients; pooled intestinal parasite prevalence reported at 28.42%, with higher prevalence in solid tumors and when culture/PCR were used.

Link: https://pmc.ncbi.nlm.nih.gov/articles/PMC12211656/

Type: Human stool-sample study **Evidence:** Prevalence evidence

Summary: 200 adult cancer patients; pathogenic intestinal parasites found in 26% of diarrheic stool samples and 15% of formed stool samples; authors recommended parasite testing/treatment before chemotherapy in high-prevalence settings.

Link: https://pubmed.ncbi.nlm.nih.gov/9204612/

3. Intestinal parasitic infections in patients with malignancy (1997)

Type: Retrospective study **Evidence:** Prevalence evidence

Summary: 1,029 cancer patients with diarrhea; intestinal parasites were found in 16.5% of cases; many had hematopoietic cancers and were receiving chemotherapy.

Link: https://pubmed.ncbi.nlm.nih.gov/9360344/

4. Prevalence and molecular identification of protozoan intestinal parasitic infections in cancer patients and a control group (2024)

Type: Case-control / molecular study **Evidence:** Moderate prevalence evidence

Summary: Iran study: protozoan infections were higher in cancer patients than controls, reported as 31.6% vs 12.0%; Blastocystis was common.

Link: https://pmc.ncbi.nlm.nih.gov/articles/PMC11603904/

5. Study on intestinal parasitic infections and gut microbiota in cancer patients at a tertiary teaching hospital in Malaysia (2024)

Type: Cancer patient/control study **Evidence:** Moderate prevalence evidence

Summary: Scientific Reports study reporting intestinal parasite infections in Malaysian cancer patients, with Microsporidia frequently detected and none detected in healthy controls in the study.

Link: https://www.nature.com/articles/s41598-024-59969-6

6. Prevalence of Intestinal Helminths among Cancer Patients Who Are under Chemotherapy (2022)

Type: Cross-sectional study **Evidence:** Prevalence evidence

Summary: Ethiopia study of cancer patients undergoing chemotherapy; reported intestinal helminth infections including hookworm, Ascaris, and Hymenolepis nana.

Link: https://pmc.ncbi.nlm.nih.gov/articles/PMC9038382/

7. Intestinal parasites in cancer patients in the South of Brazil (2018)

Type: Cross-sectional study **Evidence:** Prevalence evidence

Summary: Study of intestinal parasites in cancer patients undergoing chemotherapy in southern Brazil; relevant to chemo/immunosuppression risk.

Link: https://www.scielo.br/j/bjb/a/VzgL4QNGM69M3QsSQNSxjSs/?format=html&lang=en

8. Prevalence of Intestinal Parasitic Infection in Cancer, Organ Transplant, and Primary Immunodeficiency Patients (2019)

Type: Comparative immunocompromised-patient study **Evidence:** Prevalence evidence

Summary: Reported intestinal parasites in cancer patients and other immunocompromised groups; Blastocystis was prominent among cancer patients.

Link: https://hero.epa.gov/reference/6187077/

9. Intestinal Parasites Infection in Children with Cancer in Ahvaz, Southwest Iran (2020)

Type: Pediatric cancer study **Evidence:** Prevalence evidence

Summary: Study reported parasitic infections in 35.9% of children with cancer, including Giardia, Entamoeba coli, Blastocystis, and others.

Link: https://pmc.ncbi.nlm.nih.gov/articles/PMC7775128/

10. Intestinal parasitism in pediatric oncology children receiving chemotherapy (2019)

Type: Pediatric oncology study **Evidence:** Prevalence evidence / lower rate

Summary: Study of pediatric oncology patients; overall enteroparasite prevalence was 6.6%, showing that rates vary widely by region/testing/population.

Link: https://pmc.ncbi.nlm.nih.gov/articles/PMC6702426/

11. Protozoan Intestinal Parasitic Infection in Patients with Hematological Malignancies (2022)

Type: Hematologic malignancy study **Evidence:** Prevalence evidence

Summary: Study evaluating gastrointestinal protozoan infection frequency in patients with hematological malignancies undergoing intensive treatment.

Link: https://www.mdpi.com/2077-0383/11/10/2847

Pancreatic-specific

1. A Case of Concurrence of Clonorchis Sinensis and Pancreatic Adenocarcinoma—A Diagnostic Dilemma (2023)

Type: Case report **Evidence:** Case report only

Summary: 80-year-old man with pancreatic adenocarcinoma associated with Clonorchis sinensis infection; important pancreatic-specific coexistence case, not proof of causation.

Link: https://pmc.ncbi.nlm.nih.gov/articles/PMC9924632/

2. Small pancreatic cancer with giardiasis: a case report (2010)

Type: Case report **Evidence:** Case report only

Summary: Pancreatic cancer case with Giardia infection; documents coexistence but does not establish Giardia as the cause.

Link: https://pubmed.ncbi.nlm.nih.gov/20664486/

3. Another case of coincidental Giardia infection and pancreatic cancer (2019)

Type: Case report **Evidence:** Case report only / likely coincidental

Summary: Giardia infection coexisting with pancreatic cancer; authors describe the relationship as coincidental and note only a few such cases.

Link: https://pubmed.ncbi.nlm.nih.gov/31002881/

4. Giardia-filled Pancreatic Mass in a Patient With Recently Treated T-cell-rich B-cell Lymphoma (2017)

Summary: Reported a Giardia-filled pancreatic cystic mass; supports the point that parasites can create or occupy pancreatic mass-like lesions.

Link: https://pmc.ncbi.nlm.nih.gov/articles/PMC5346013/

5. A case of human pancreatic eurytremiasis (2019)

Type: Case report/imaging **Evidence:** Case report only

Summary: Human pancreatic eurytremiasis with pancreatic/biliary findings; useful for pancreatic parasite differential diagnosis.

Link: https://pubmed.ncbi.nlm.nih.gov/30758533/

Pancreatic-specific / autopsy

1. Human infection with the pancreas fluke, Eurytrema pancreaticum (1983)

Type: Autopsy case report **Evidence:** Autopsy evidence

Summary: 70-year-old Japanese woman with gastric cancer found at autopsy to have about 15 adult Eurytrema pancreaticum flukes in dilated pancreatic ducts. Proves a cancer patient had pancreatic flukes at autopsy; does not prove causation.

Link: https://pubmed.ncbi.nlm.nih.gov/6625056/

Pancreatic-specific / mimic

1. Primary pancreatic hydatid cyst: A rare case report and diagnostic challenges (2024)

Type: Case report **Evidence:** Tumor mimic case report

Summary: Primary pancreatic hydatid cyst caused by Echinococcus granulosus, challenging to diagnose and capable of mimicking pancreatic cystic neoplasm.

Link: https://pmc.ncbi.nlm.nih.gov/articles/PMC11230916/

2. Primary pancreatic hydatid cyst misdiagnosed as pancreatic cystic neoplasm (2021)

Type: Case report **Evidence:** Tumor mimic case report

Summary: Report/review of pancreatic hydatid cyst that can be misdiagnosed as pancreatic cystic neoplasm; supports careful differential diagnosis before major treatment.

Link: https://link.springer.com/article/10.1186/s12876-021-01753-1

3. Acute pancreatitis revealing an isolated hydatid cyst of the pancreas (2023)

Type: Case report **Evidence:** Tumor mimic case report

Summary: Pancreatic hydatid cyst is described as rare and widely misdiagnosed, especially as an isolated cystic lesion simulating a pancreatic lesion.

Link: https://europepmc.org/article/pmc/pmc10017306

4. Report of an undiagnosed case of pancreatic hydatid cyst and brief literature review (2014)

Type: Case report/review **Evidence:** Tumor mimic case report

Summary: Notes that pancreatic hydatid cyst is rare, can cause pancreato-biliary complications, and preoperative diagnosis is challenging.

Link: https://www.wjgnet.com/1948-9366/full/v6/i10/190.htm

Pancreatic-specific / diagnosis

1. Mayo Clinic – Pancreatic cancer diagnosis and treatment (Current)

Type: Clinical information page **Evidence:** Clinical background

Summary: Explains pancreatic cancer diagnostic workup including biopsy/tissue sampling; useful to support the need for diagnostic confirmation before treatment when appropriate.

Link: https://www.mayoclinic.org/diseases-conditions/pancreatic-cancer/diagnosis-treatment/drc-20355427

Tumor mimic / pathology

1. Colonic schistosomiasis mimicking cancer, polyp, and inflammatory bowel disease: five case reports and review (2024)

Type: Case series/review **Evidence:** Tumor mimic evidence

Summary: Five cases of intestinal schistosomiasis mimicking cancer, polyps, or inflammatory bowel disease; supports parasite mimicry differential diagnosis.

Link: https://pmc.ncbi.nlm.nih.gov/articles/PMC11325876/

2. Strongyloides stercoralis infection mimicking a malignant tumour (2005)

Type: Case report **Evidence:** Tumor mimic evidence

Summary: Fatal strongyloidiasis in an older patient presenting in a way that mimicked malignant disease.

Link: https://pmc.ncbi.nlm.nih.gov/articles/PMC1770632/

3. Leishmania infantum mimicking lymphoma in an elderly patient (2023)

Type: Case report **Evidence:** Tumor mimic evidence

Summary: Case of Leishmania presenting as a lesion mimicking lymphoma; relevant to differential diagnosis of malignancy-like lesions.

Link: https://pmc.ncbi.nlm.nih.gov/articles/PMC10162717/

4. Echinococcosis/hydatid disease mimicking malignancy (2018)

Type: Case report/review **Evidence:** Tumor mimic evidence

Summary: Hydatid disease can mimic malignancy or metastasis in organs such as liver/lung/bone; supports infectious differential diagnosis.

Link: https://pmc.ncbi.nlm.nih.gov/articles/PMC5793748/

5. Huge colonic granuloma of schistosomiasis mimicked cancer in a 10-year-old child (2022)

Type: Case report **Evidence:** Tumor mimic evidence

Summary: Schistosomiasis-associated colonic granuloma mimicked cancer; diagnosis confirmed by histopathology of resected mass.

Link: https://www.dovepress.com/huge-colonic-granuloma-of-schistosomiasis-mimicked-cancer-in-a-10-year-peer-reviewed-

6. Hepatic pseudotumor associated with Strongyloides infection (2023)

Type: Case report **Evidence:** Tumor mimic evidence

Summary: Strongyloides-associated hepatic pseudotumor showed radiographic similarity to malignant liver tumors, raising risk of misdiagnosis and invasive interventions.

Link: https://www.wjgnet.com/1948-5182/full/v15/i12/1338.htm

Autopsy / cancer patients with parasites

1. Strongyloides stercoralis hyperinfection discovered at autopsy in a patient with multiple myeloma (2008)

Type: Autopsy case report **Evidence:** Autopsy evidence

Summary: Autopsy case in a patient treated for multiple myeloma; supports that parasites can be found in cancer/immunosuppressed patients and can cause fatal hyperinfection.

Link: https://pubmed.ncbi.nlm.nih.gov/18853018/

2. Disseminated strongyloidiasis: study of seven autopsy cases (1994)

Type: Autopsy series **Evidence:** Autopsy evidence

Summary: Autopsy series of disseminated strongyloidiasis in immunosuppressed patients, relevant to cancer/chemotherapy risk contexts.

Link: https://pubmed.ncbi.nlm.nih.gov/8058699/

3. Cysticercosis and neoplasia: an autopsy study (2013)

Type: Autopsy study **Evidence:** Coexistence evidence

Summary: Autopsy-based study examining coexistence of cysticercosis and neoplasia. Useful but does not prove cysticercosis caused the cancers.

Link: https://pmc.ncbi.nlm.nih.gov/articles/PMC3830783/

Other parasite-cancer associations

1. Toxoplasma gondii infection/exposure and risk of brain tumors: systematic review/meta-analysis (2022)

Type: Systematic review/meta-analysis **Evidence:** Suggestive / not proven causal

Summary: Provides suggestive evidence for an association between T. gondii exposure and brain tumors/glioma; causation not proven.

Link: https://pubmed.ncbi.nlm.nih.gov/35152168/

2. Is there association between Trichomonas vaginalis infection and prostate cancer risk? A systematic review and meta-analysis (2019)

Type: Systematic review/meta-analysis **Evidence:** Mixed/limited

Summary: Evaluates the possible association between Trichomonas vaginalis infection and prostate cancer risk; evidence is mixed and not definitive.

Link: https://pubmed.ncbi.nlm.nih.gov/31539586/

Type: Cohort/serology analysis **Evidence:** Contradictory/limiting evidence

Summary: Found no association between T. vaginalis serostatus and prostate cancer mortality or all-cause mortality in studied cohorts.

Link: https://pmc.ncbi.nlm.nih.gov/articles/PMC6430694/

4. Trichomonas vaginalis infection and risk of advanced prostate cancer (2016)

Type: Nested case-control / cohort analysis **Evidence:** Contradictory/limiting evidence

Summary: Study did not support increased risk of advanced or fatal prostate cancer among men seropositive for T. vaginalis.

Link: https://pubmed.ncbi.nlm.nih.gov/26818005/

5. Are Blastocystis hominis and Cryptosporidium spp. playing a positive role in colorectal cancer risk? (2022)

Type: Systematic review/meta-analysis **Evidence:** Weak/moderate association

Summary: Systematic review/meta-analysis of Blastocystis and Cryptosporidium prevalence/odds in colorectal cancer; association studied, causation not proven.

Link: https://pmc.ncbi.nlm.nih.gov/articles/PMC9206311/

6. Role of Cryptosporidium spp. in Development of Colorectal Cancer (2023)

Type: Case-control/observational study **Evidence:** Emerging/association

Summary: Study of cryptosporidiosis among colorectal cancer patients compared with healthy subjects; supports further research but not definitive causation.

Link: https://pmc.ncbi.nlm.nih.gov/articles/PMC10162599/

7. Cryptosporidium and Colon Cancer: Cause or Consequence? (2020)

Type: Review **Evidence:** Exploratory/mechanistic review

Summary: Review discussing potential causal links between Cryptosporidium infection and digestive cancer, especially colon cancer.

Link: https://pmc.ncbi.nlm.nih.gov/articles/PMC7692234/

8. Association of Blastocystis hominis with colorectal cancer (2022)

Type: Systematic review **Evidence:** Association / not causation

Summary: Review of studies on Blastocystis prevalence in colorectal cancer patients; association reported in some studies but causality is unresolved.

Link: https://pmc.ncbi.nlm.nih.gov/articles/PMC8919012/

9. The associated risk of Blastocystis infection in cancer (2023)

Type: Observational/molecular study **Evidence:** Association / not causation

Summary: Study assessing possible association between Blastocystis infection and cancer, especially colorectal cancer, including subtype considerations.

Link: https://www.frontiersin.org/journals/oncology/articles/10.3389/fonc.2023.1115835/full

10. Colorectal Cancer Related to Chronic Strongyloides stercoralis Infection (2020)

Type: Case vignette/report **Evidence:** Case report only

Summary: Case involving chronic Strongyloides infection and colorectal cancer; useful as a case-level association, not proof of general causation.

Link: https://pmc.ncbi.nlm.nih.gov/articles/PMC7492975/

Antiparasitic drug / cancer research

1. Johns Hopkins – Anti-parasitic drug slows pancreatic cancer in mice (2021)

Type: Institutional research summary **Evidence:** Animal/preclinical

Summary: Johns Hopkins summary of mebendazole research showing slowed pancreatic cancer initiation/progression/metastasis in mouse models; not proof of human efficacy.

Link: https://www.hopkinsmedicine.org/news/newsroom/news-releases/2021/08/johns-hopkins-study-anti-parasitic-drug-slows-pancreatic-cancer-in-mice

2. Ivermectin and gemcitabine combination suppresses pancreatic cancer in preclinical models (2022)

Type: Lab/animal study **Evidence:** Preclinical only

Summary: Study found ivermectin plus gemcitabine suppressed pancreatic cancer cells and tumor growth in lab/mouse models; not proof that ivermectin treats human pancreatic cancer.

Link: https://pubmed.ncbi.nlm.nih.gov/36091811/

3. American Cancer Society – What to Know About Ivermectin and Cancer (2026)

Type: Cancer organization guidance **Evidence:** Clinical caution / limitation

Summary: States ivermectin is not approved to treat cancer and no clinical guidelines recommend it as cancer treatment; useful limiting source.

Link: https://www.cancer.org/cancer/latest-news/what-to-know-about-ivermectin.html

4. ASCO Clinical Notice recommending against ivermectin and fenbendazole for cancer treatment (2026)

Type: Professional oncology guidance **Evidence:** Clinical caution / limitation

Summary: ASCO clinical notice cautioning against ivermectin and fenbendazole as cancer treatment or adjuncts outside evidence-based care.

Link: https://connection.asco.org/do/asco-clinical-notice-recommending-against-ivermectin-and-fenbendazole-cancer-treatment

Spontaneous regression context

1. Spontaneous regression of cancer: review / immune mechanisms (2021)

Type: Review **Evidence:** Context source

Summary: Discusses rare spontaneous regression/remission of cancer and possible mechanisms such as immune activation, infection, fever, apoptosis, or tumor ischemia; not proof of parasite death.

Link: https://pmc.ncbi.nlm.nih.gov/articles/PMC8271173/

2. Spontaneous regression of metastatic pancreatic cancer case report/review (2019)

Summary: Documents rare spontaneous regression in pancreatic cancer context; possible immune mechanisms discussed, not proof of parasite involvement.

Link: https://pmc.ncbi.nlm.nih.gov/articles/PMC6557416/

Suggested next search terms

- parasites and cancer PubMed
- parasites found in cancer patients autopsy
- pancreatic cancer parasite case report
- parasites found in tumor tissue pathology
- Schistosoma haematobium bladder cancer IARC
- Opisthorchis viverrini cholangiocarcinoma IARC
- Clonorchis sinensis cholangiocarcinoma IARC
- Hymenolepis nana malignant transformation human host
- intestinal parasites cancer patients chemotherapy meta-analysis
- pancreatic hydatid cyst mimicking neoplasm

www.ingramcontent.com/pod-product-compliance
Lightning Source LLC
LaVergne TN
LVHW080022210926
848481LV00011B/3081